Alcoholic/Non-Alcoholic Digestive Diseases

Hitoshi Yoshiji • Kosuke Kaji
Editors

Alcoholic/Non-Alcoholic Digestive Diseases

Springer

Editors
Hitoshi Yoshiji
Third Department of Internal Medicine
Nara Medical University
Kashihara
Japan

Kosuke Kaji
Third Department of Internal Medicine
Nara Medical University
Kashihara
Japan

ISBN 978-981-13-1464-3 ISBN 978-981-13-1465-0 (eBook)
https://doi.org/10.1007/978-981-13-1465-0

This Springer imprint is published by the registered company Springer Nature Singapore Pte Ltd.
The registered company address is: 152 Beach Road, #21-01/04 Gateway East, Singapore 189721, Singapore

Preface

Over the last decade, there has been an explosion in understanding the treatment of alcoholic/non-alcoholic digestive diseases as well as various clinical challenges and research results. Alcohol, nutrition, and dietary habits are closely related to most lifestyle-related diseases as well as people's quality of life. These lead to not only ischemic heart disease but also digestive system disorders. Alcohol confers a direct impact on the digestive system due to its contact with gastrointestinal mucosa and disturbance in digestive functions. Various diseases of the gastrointestinal tract may be associated with an excessive alcohol intake, and the relationship between alcohol consumption and hepatic and pancreatic damage is widely recognized. Obesity-based metabolic syndrome has been seen as a risk factor for a variety of digestive diseases, and obesity has been implicated in various gastrointestinal diseases including gastroesophageal reflex diseases and colorectal cancer as well as liver diseases known as non-alcoholic fatty liver diseases.

The aim of this book is to bring together in one place reviews of the several different fields. In this book, Part I (Chaps. 1–5) consists of the clinical and basic insights of alcoholic/non-alcoholic gastrointestinal diseases and includes the chapters "Alcohol and esophageal cancer" (Chap. 1), "Gastroesophageal reflex disease in metabolic syndrome" (Chap. 2), "*H. pylori*-negative gastric diseases" (Chaps. 3 and 4), and "Alcohol and metabolic diseases in colorectal cancer" (Chap. 5). Part II (Chaps. 6–11) highlights liver diseases. This part introduces various key players in the pathophysiology of alcoholic liver injury and non-alcoholic fatty liver diseases, including "Extracellular vesicles" (Chap. 6), "Diabetes mellitus" (Chap. 7), "Obesity" (Chap. 8), "Microbiota" (Chap. 9), "Oxidative stress" (Chap. 10), and "Apoptosis" (Chap. 11). Finally, in Part III (Chaps. 12 and 13), new perspectives in pancreatic diseases including "Alcohol and chronic pancreatitis" (Chap. 12) and "New therapeutics in pancreatic cancer" (Chap. 13) are provided. Taken together, this book provides excellent coverage of the current knowledge of molecular mechanism, therapeutic application, and will be of great interest to leading scientists on the cutting-edge of alcoholic/non-alcoholic digestive diseases.

Finally, we would like to thank all of the authors for their contributions as well as Springer Japan for their efforts in publishing this book.

Kashihara, Japan Hitoshi Yoshiji
Kashihara, Japan Kosuke Kaji

Contents

Part I
Alcoholic/Non-Alcoholic Gastrointestinal Diseases

Chapter 1
Alcohol-Induced DNA Injury in Esophageal Squamous Cell Carcinoma

Masashi Tamaoki, Yusuke Amanuma, Shinya Ohashi, and Manabu Muto

Abstract Alcohol consumption is a major risk factor for esophageal squamous cell carcinoma. Acetaldehyde, a highly reactive compound that causes various types of DNA damage, plays a central role in alcohol-induced esophageal carcinogenesis. Acetaldehyde is mainly generated from the metabolism of ethanol by alcohol dehydrogenase 1B and is then detoxified to acetic acid by aldehyde dehydrogenase 2 (ALDH2). Alcohol consumption increases blood, saliva, and breath acetaldehyde levels, especially in individuals with inactive ALDH2 that are strongly associated with the risk of squamous cell carcinoma in the esophagus. In this chapter, we review recent studies of alcohol-mediated carcinogenesis in the squamous epithelium of the esophagus, focusing especially on acetaldehyde-induced DNA damage.

Keywords Acetaldehyde · DNA damage · DNA adduct

1.1 Acetaldehyde, a Metabolite of Alcohol, and the Development of Esophageal Squamous Cell Carcinoma

Esophageal cancer is the eighth most common cancer worldwide [1]. There are two main histological subtypes of esophageal cancer: esophageal squamous cell carcinoma (ESCC) and esophageal adenocarcinoma, the incidence of which varies between regions [1]. Alcohol consumption has been shown to be a risk factor for ESCC, but not for esophageal adenocarcinoma [2]. Epidemiologically, ESCC is most prevalent in Eastern Asia, Eastern and Southern Africa, and Southern Europe [3, 4]. These variations suggest that the incidence of ESCC is affected by genetic

M. Tamaoki · Y. Amanuma · S. Ohashi · M. Muto (✉)
Department of Therapeutic Oncology, Graduate School of Medicine, Kyoto University, Kyoto, Japan
e-mail: tamaoki@kuhp.kyoto-u.ac.jp; yusuke12@kuhp.kyoto-u.ac.jp; ohashish@kuhp.kyoto-u.ac.jp; mmuto@kuhp.kyoto-u.ac.jp

H. Yoshiji, K. Kaji (eds.), *Alcoholic/Non-Alcoholic Digestive Diseases*,
https://doi.org/10.1007/978-981-13-1465-0_1

differences between races. These genetic differences and/or alcohol consumption are thought to be involved in esophageal carcinogenesis via generation of acetaldehyde, a highly reactive compound that causes DNA damage [5, 6].

Ingested ethanol in alcohol beverage is primarily absorbed from the upper gastrointestinal tract and transported to the liver, where it is mainly metabolized into acetaldehyde by cytosolic alcohol dehydrogenase 1B (ADH1B). Acetaldehyde is then detoxified to acetic acid by mitochondrial aldehyde dehydrogenase 2 (ALDH2) (Fig. 1.1a) [7, 8]. The *ADH1B* gene is on chromosome 4 and has two major alleles: *ADH1B*1* (less active ADH1B) and *ADH1B*2* (active ADH1B, rs1229984) (Fig. 1.1b). The rs1229984 allele (*ADH1B*2*) of *ADH1B*, known as Arg48His, encodes an ADH1B protein that mediates a high clearance rate of ethanol from the liver. There are three genotypes of ADH1B: *ADH1B*1/*1* (less active, slow metabolizing ADH1B); *ADH1B*1/*2* and *ADH1B*2/*2* (active ADH1B) [9]. Meta-analysis has revealed that individuals with *ADH1B*1/*1* have a 2.77-times higher risk of ESCC [10] and a 2.35-times higher risk of head and neck squamous cell carcinoma (HNSCC) [11] compared with individuals with the *ADH1B*1* allele (*ADH1B*1/*2* and *ADH1B*2/*2*). The frequency of the *ADH1B*1* allele is much higher in ethnic populations from Europe, America, and Africa than in those from East Asia, while *ADH1B*2* is the major allele present in East Asia [12].

The *ALDH2* gene is on chromosome 12 and has two major alleles: *ALDH2*1* (active ALDH2) and *ALDH2*2* (inactive ALDH2, rs671) (Fig. 1.1b). The rs671 allele (*ALDH2*2*) of *ALDH2* encodes an ALDH2 protein that is defective at metabolizing acetaldehyde; this single nucleotide polymorphism is also known as Glu504Lys. As *ALDH2*2* acts in a dominant negative manner, a phenotypic loss of ALDH2 activity is seen in both heterozygous (*ALDH2*1/*2*) and homozygous (*ALDH2*2/*2*) genotypes [13]. Therefore, ALDH2 is divided into three genotypes: *ALDH2*1/*1*, active (100% activity) ALDH2; *ALDH2*1/*2*, inactive (<10% activity) ALDH2; and *ALDH2*2/*2*, inactive (0% activity) ALDH2 [14]. The *ALDH2*2* allele (rs671) is prevalent in Asian [15], and carriers of the *ALDH2*2* allele account for about 40% of East Asian populations [16]. Heavy alcohol consumption increases the risk of ESCC in people with the *ALDH2*2* polymorphism [17], which could account for the higher incidence of ESCC in Asian versus Western countries [7]. Meta-analysis has shown that individuals with *ALDH2*1/*2* have a 7.12-times higher risk of ESCC [18] and a 1.83-times higher risk of HNSCC [19] compared with individuals with *ALDH2*1/*1*. Moreover, alcoholics with the *ALDH2*1/*2* genotype have a 13.5-times higher risk of ESCC and an 18.52-times higher risk of HNSCC compared with alcoholics with *ALDH2*1/*1* [20]. According to a recent study, individuals with either the *ADH1B*1* or *ALDH2*2* allele have a risk of alcohol-mediated gene mutations in ESCC [21].

In addition to "endogenous" acetaldehyde produced from alcohol metabolism, acetaldehyde can also be produced by microorganisms in the oral cavity [22, 23]. Moreover, acetaldehyde is contained as "free" acetaldehyde in foods such as yogurt, ripe fruits, cheese, coffee, and alcoholic beverages [24, 25], as well as in tobacco smoke [26]. Notably, some alcoholic beverages such as Calvados contain

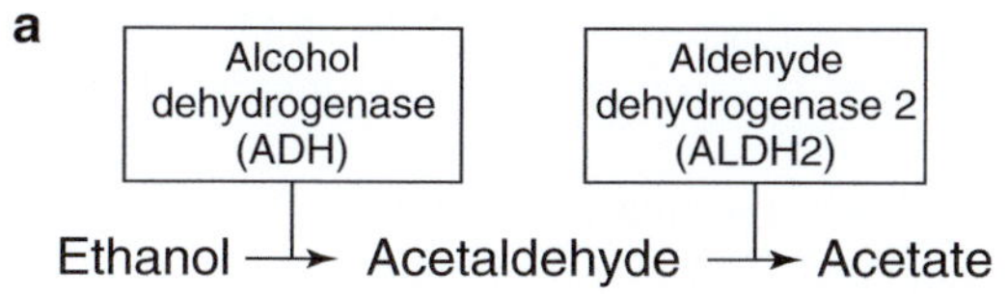

b

Gene	rs	Cytogenetic location	Genomic location (on assembly GRCh38)	Reference allele	Alternate allele	amino acid transition
ADH1B	1229984	4q23	Chr4: 99318162	G	A	Arg48His
ALDH2	671	12q24	Chr12: 111803962	G	A	Glu504Lys

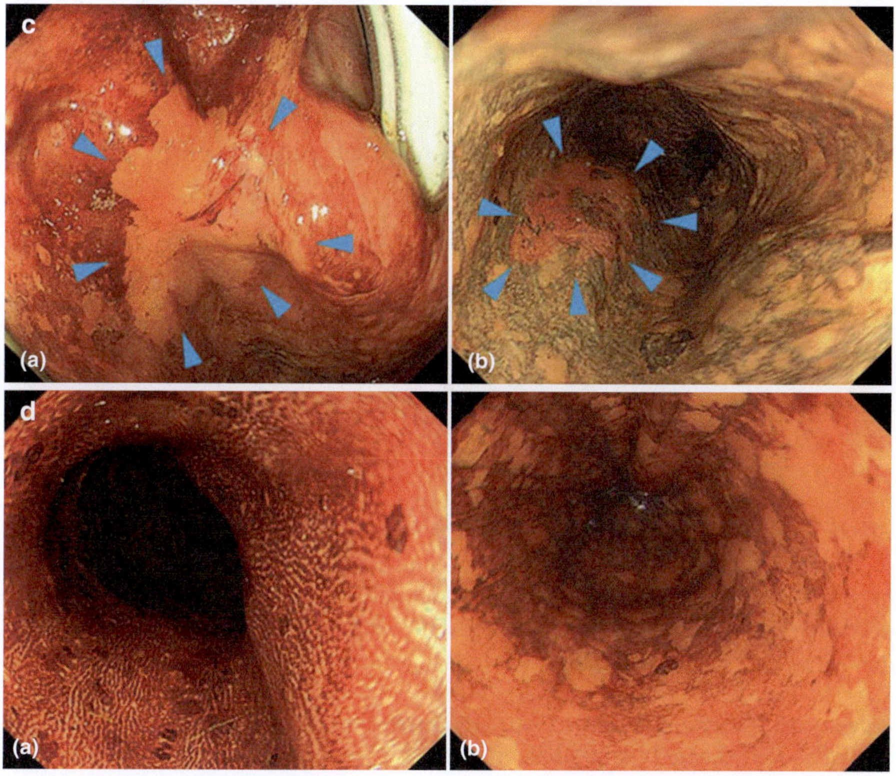

Fig. 1.1 Alcohol metabolism and Lugol-chromoendoscopy images. (**a**) Metabolism of ethanol and acetaldehyde. Ethanol is metabolized into acetaldehyde by ADH1B, and acetaldehyde is then detoxified to acetic acid by ALDH2. (**b**) Summary of the major single-nucleotide polymorphisms (SNPs) in the *ADH1B* and *ALDH2* genes. The rs1229984 allele of *ADH1B* (*ADH1B*2*) encodes a form of active ADH1B protein that increases the metabolism of ethanol. The rs671 allele of the *ALDH2* (*ALDH2*2*) encodes a form of inactive ALDH2 protein that is defective at metabolizing acetaldehyde. rs: reference single nucleotide polymorphism ID number. (**c**) Lugol-endoscopic images of "field cancerization" in a patient with synchronous squamous cell carcinomas in the oropharynx (*a*) and middle thoracic esophagus (*b*). Lesions are indicated by arrowheads; (**d**) Lugol-endoscopic images of normal esophageal mucosa (*a*), and esophageal mucosa with multiple dysplasia recognized as multiple Lugol-voiding lesions (*b*)

very high quantities of free acetaldehyde (e.g., calvados: 1781 ± 861 μM), and habitual consumption of these beverages is associated with an increased risk of ESCC [27].

Based on this epidemiological evidence, the International Agency for Research on Cancer defined acetaldehyde associated with alcohol intake as a "group 1 carcinogen" for esophagus, and head and neck [28].

ESCC also occurs synchronously and/or metachronously in conjunction with HNSCC; this phenomenon has been recognized as "field cancerization" [29] (Fig. 1.1c). Squamous dysplasia is a preneoplastic lesion of ESCC that can be visualized by Lugol chromoendoscopy as multiple Lugol-voiding lesions (LVLs) (Fig. 1.1d) [30, 31]. A recent prospective cohort study revealed that the severity of LVLs is associated with average alcohol consumption, and that patients with severe multiple LVLs are at significantly higher risk for the development of metachronous multiple ESCC and HNSCC [32]. Of note, the *ALDH2*2* allele is the strongest contributing factor (OR: 17.6) for the development of multiple LVLs [33]. Thus, alcohol consumption in individuals with the *ALDH2*2* allele and/or multiple LVLs in their background mucosa is associated with a high risk of "field cancerization."

1.2 Blood and Saliva Acetaldehyde Concentration After Alcohol Intake

Alcohol intake increases blood, saliva, and breath levels of acetaldehyde [33, 34]. In particular, acetaldehyde reaches high concentrations in saliva compared with blood [22]. When individuals drink 0.6 g ethanol/kg body weight, acetaldehyde concentrations in saliva rapidly reach 24–53 μM in *ALDH2*1/*1* carriers compared with 37–76 μM in *ALDH2*1/*2* carriers, while blood acetaldehyde concentrations are 2–5 μM in *ALDH2*1/*1* carriers and 12–25 μM in *ALDH2*1/*2* carriers [35].

Local microbial and/or mucosal acetaldehyde production in the oral cavity and acetaldehyde secretion from salivary glands are considered to play a role in the carcinogenesis of alcohol-related upper gastrointestinal tract cancers [7, 36, 37]. In the oral cavity, *Streptococcus* is the most abundant bacterial genus, followed by *Haemophilus*, *Neisseria*, *Prevotella*, *Veillonella,* and *Rothia* [38]. *Neisseria* and *Streptococcus* species can produce mutagenic levels of acetaldehyde from ethanol in vitro [23, 39]. In addition, fungal flora, including the *Candida* genus, contribute to acetaldehyde generation [40, 41]. Secretion from salivary glands also influences the acetaldehyde level in saliva, because alcohol consumption significantly increases the acetaldehyde concentration in the parotid-duct saliva of *ALDH2*1/*2* carriers compared with that of *ALDH2*1/*1* carriers [42]. Acetaldehyde in the breath is also thought to dissolve into the saliva [43].

Overall, these data indicate that alcohol consumption by *ALDH2*1/*2* carriers could result in the direct exposure of the mucosa of the pharynx and esophagus to saliva containing sustained high levels of acetaldehyde.

1.3 Acetaldehyde Reacts with DNA to Form DNA Adducts and Cause Severe DNA Damage

Although the precise mechanism of acetaldehyde-mediated esophageal carcinogenesis has been unknown, DNA damage caused by acetaldehyde is thought to be involved in esophageal carcinogenesis [43]. Acetaldehyde is strongly electrophilic and can therefore react directly with DNA, especially with the exocyclic amino group of deoxyguanosine (dG). This reaction results in the formation of DNA adducts such as N^2-ethylidene-2′-deoxyguanosine (N^2-ethylidene-dG) [44], N^2-ethyl-2′-deoxyguanosine (N^2-Et-dG) [45], -S- and -R-methyl-hydroxy-1,N^2-propano-2′-deoxyguanosine (CrPdG), and 1,N^2-etheno-2′-deoxyguanosine (NεG) (Fig. 1.2a) [44, 46].

N^2-ethylidene-dG, the major DNA adduct derived from acetaldehyde, is generated from a single molecule of acetaldehyde and dG [47]. Alcohol consumption increases oral and blood N^2-ethylidene-dG levels [48, 49] to a degree that is associated with the *ALDH2* genotype [50]. Blood N^2-ethylidene-dG levels in alcoholics with the *ALDH2*2* allele are higher than in those with the *ALDH2*1/*1* allele [51]. Alcohol consumption also increases the "esophageal" levels of N^2-ethylidene-dG in *Aldh2*-knockout mice compared with wild-type mice [49, 52]. N^2-Et-dG blocks DNA synthesis and induces DNA mutations [53, 54], and also inhibits translesional DNA synthesis, which results in frameshift deletions and G:C > T:A transversions [54].

Two molecules of acetaldehyde can be converted into crotonaldehyde, which then reacts with DNA to form CrPdG [55]. The CrPdG level is closely related to the amount of acetaldehyde produced [56]. CrPdG exists in both ring-opened and ring-closed forms [57, 58]. CrPdG causes DNA interstrand [59] and intrastrand cross-links [60]. The ring-opened form of CrPdG reacts with dG on the opposite strand of the DNA and forms DNA interstrand cross-links [61]; DNA intrastrand cross-links are mediated by a similar mechanism [6]. The ring-closed form of CrPdG would be incapable of Watson–Crick base pairing with cytosine in the anti-conformation, but Hoogsteen base pairing with cytosine would be possible in the syn-conformation [58]. Such CrPdG-mediated disruption of the DNA replication process is thought to result in DNA damage [58].

NεG is generated from 2′-deoxyguanosine and α,β-unsaturated aldehydes, which can be formed during lipid peroxidation mediated by acetaldehyde [55, 62]. When acetaldehyde induces the generation of reactive oxygen species (ROS) leading to lipid peroxidation [63], generation of NεG can be mediated by acetaldehyde and/or ROS. NεG induces mutations such as base-pair mutations, deletions, rearrangements and DNA double-strand breaks [6, 64].

Acetaldehyde exposure increases the rates of sister chromatid exchange (SCE) in human cells [65], although the adducts or cross-links involved in the formation of SCEs are not known.

Overall, the accumulation of these genetic abnormalities is considered to be involved in cancer development (Fig. 1.2b). Exposure of human cells to acetaldehyde induces functional mutations, most frequently G:C > A:T transitions in the *TP53* gene [66]. The ratio of these mutations is similar to the patterns of gene variation detected in ESCC [67, 68] and HNSCC [69].

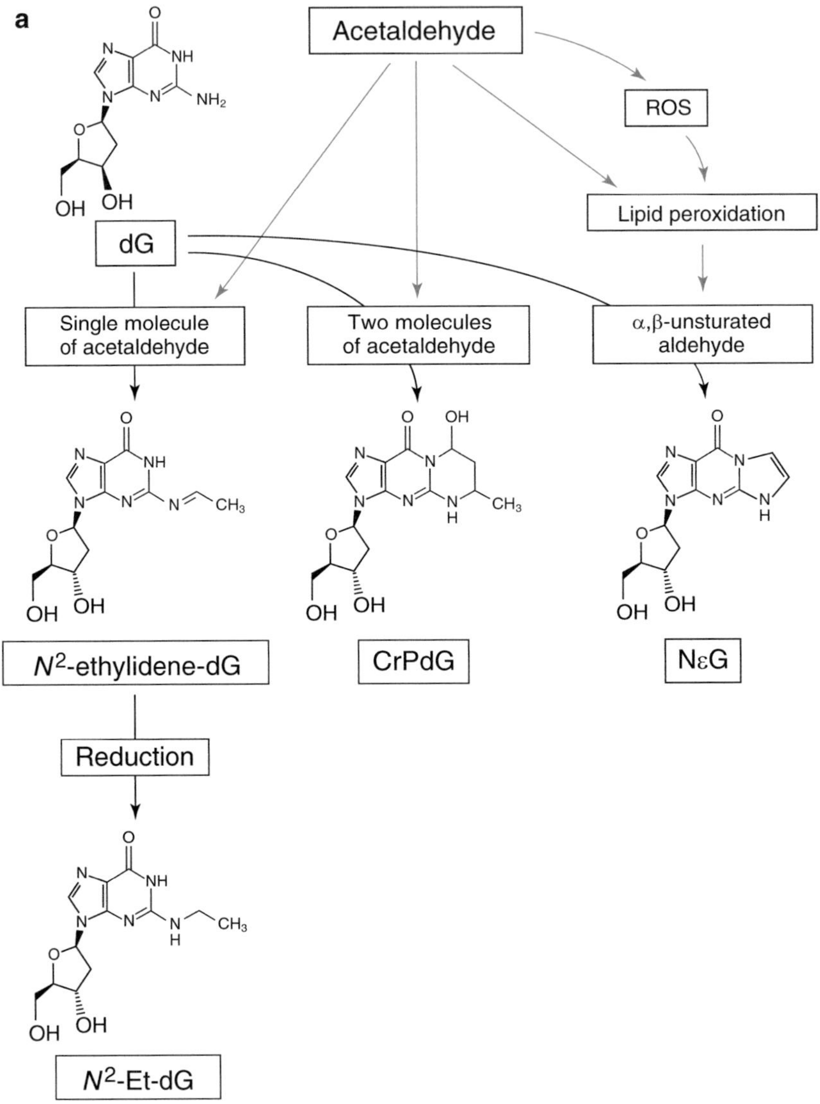

Fig. 1.2 Formation of acetaldehyde-derived DNA adducts and acetaldehyde-derived DNA damage. (**a**) A single molecule of acetaldehyde reacts directly with deoxyguanosine (dG) to form N^2-ethylidene-2′-deoxyguanosine (N^2-ethylidene-dG), which is reduced to N^2-ethyl-2′-deoxyguanosine (N^2-Et-dG). dG and two molecules of acetaldehyde form -S- and -R-methyl-hydroxy-1,N^2-propano-2′-deoxyguanosine (CrPdG). N^2-etheno-2′-deoxyguanosine (NεG) is generated from dG and α,β-unsaturated aldehydes formed during lipid peroxidation, which is triggered by acetaldehyde and/or reactive oxygen species (ROS). (**b**) Acetaldehyde induces DNA adducts, DNA single-strand breaks, point mutations, micronucleus, frameshift mutations, double-strand breaks, sister chromatid exchanges, DNA interstrand and intrastrand cross-links, base pair mutations, deletions and rearrangements

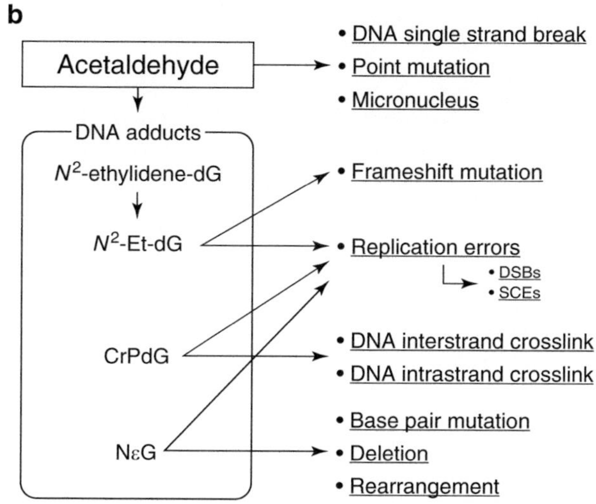

Fig. 1.2 (continued)

1.4 Conclusions

- Alcohol ingestion is a risk factor for ESCC, especially in individuals with the *ALDH2*2* allele. Acetaldehyde is strongly suggested to be involved in the pathophysiology of ESCC.
- Acetaldehyde production related to alcohol metabolism and local acetaldehyde production in the oral cavity are thought to be centrally involved in esophageal carcinogenesis.
- Acetaldehyde induces various forms of DNA damage leading to cancer development, and DNA adduct formation is thought to be important for esophageal carcinogenesis.

References

1. Torre LA, et al. Global cancer statistics, 2012. CA Cancer J Clin. 2015;65:87–108.
2. Pennathur A, et al. Oesophageal carcinoma. Lancet. 2013;381:400–12.
3. Pickens A, et al. Geographical distribution and racial disparity in esophageal cancer. Ann Thorac Surg. 2003;76:S1367–9.
4. Bosetti C, et al. Trends in oesophageal cancer incidence and mortality in Europe. Int J Cancer. 2008;122:1118–29.
5. Seitz HK, et al. Molecular mechanisms of alcohol-mediated carcinogenesis. Nat Rev Cancer. 2007;7:599–612.
6. Brooks PJ, et al. Acetaldehyde and the genome: beyond nuclear DNA adducts and carcinogenesis. Environ Mol Mutagen. 2014;55:77–91.
7. Ohashi S, et al. Recent advances from basic and clinical studies of esophageal squamous cell carcinoma. Gastroenterology. 2015;149:1700–15.

8. Peng GS, et al. Effect of the allelic variants of aldehyde dehydrogenase ALDH2*2 and alcohol dehydrogenase ADH1B*2 on blood acetaldehyde concentrations. Hum Genomics. 2009;3:121–7.
9. Neumark YD, et al. Alcohol dehydrogenase polymorphisms influence alcohol-elimination rates in a male Jewish population. Alcohol Clin Exp Res. 2004;28:10–4.
10. Zhang L, et al. Gene—environment interactions on the risk of esophageal cancer among Asian populations with the G48A polymorphism in the alcohol dehydrogenase-2 gene: a meta-analysis. Tumour Biol. 2014;35:4705–17.
11. Zhang Y, et al. Alcohol dehydrogenase-1B Arg47His polymorphism is associated with head and neck cancer risk in Asian: a meta-analysis. Tumour Biol. 2015;36:1023–7.
12. Treutlein J, et al. ADH1B Arg48His allele frequency map: filling in the gap for Central Europe. Biol Psychiatry. 2014;75:e15.
13. Enomoto N, Takase S, Yasuhara M, et al. Acetaldehyde metabolism in different aldehyde dehydrogenase-2 genotypes. Alcohol Clin Exp Res. 1991;15:141–4.
14. Yokoyama A, et al. Genetic polymorphisms of alcohol dehydrogense-1B and aldehyde dehydrogenase-2, alcohol flushing, mean corpuscular volume, and aerodigestive tract neoplasia in Japanese drinkers. Adv Exp Med Biol. 2015;815:265–79.
15. Goedde HW, et al. Distribution of ADH2 and ALDH2 genotypes in different populations. Hum Genet. 1992;88:344–6.
16. Harada S, et al. Aldehyde dehydrogenase deficiency as cause of facial flushing reaction to alcohol in Japanese. Lancet (Lond Engl). 1981;2:982.
17. Matsuo K, et al. Gene–environment interaction between an aldehyde dehydrogenase-2 (ALDH2) polymorphism and alcohol consumption for the risk of esophageal cancer. Carcinogenesis. 2001;22:913–6.
18. Yang SJ, et al. Relationship between genetic polymorphisms of ALDH2 and ADH1B and esophageal cancer risk: a meta-analysis. World J Gastroenterol. 2010;16:4210–20.
19. Boccia S, et al. Aldehyde dehydrogenase 2 and head and neck cancer: a meta-analysis implementing a Mendelian randomization approach. Cancer Epidemiol Biomark Prev. 2009;18:248–54.
20. Yokoyama A, et al. Alcohol and aldehyde dehydrogenase gene polymorphisms and oropharyngolaryngeal, esophageal and stomach cancers in Japanese alcoholics. Carcinogenesis. 2001;22:433–9.
21. Chang J, et al. Genomic analysis of oesophageal squamous-cell carcinoma identifies alcohol drinking-related mutation signature and genomic alterations. Nat Commun. 2017;8:15290.
22. Homann N, et al. High acetaldehyde levels in saliva after ethanol consumption: methodological aspects and pathogenetic implications. Carcinogenesis. 1997;18:1739–43.
23. Muto M, et al. Acetaldehyde production by non-pathogenic Neisseria in human oral microflora: implications for carcinogenesis in upper aerodigestive tract. Int J Cancer. 2000;88:342–50.
24. Uebelacker M, et al. Quantitative determination of acetaldehyde in foods using automated digestion with simulated gastric fluid followed by headspace gas chromatography. J Autom Methods Manag Chem. 2011;2011:907317.
25. Lachenmeier DW, et al. The role of acetaldehyde outside ethanol metabolism in the carcinogenicity of alcoholic beverages: evidence from a large chemical survey. Food Chem Toxicol. 2008;46:2903–11.
26. Salaspuro VJ, et al. Eliminating carcinogenic acetaldehyde by cysteine from saliva during smoking. Cancer Epidemiol Biomark Prev. 2006;15:146–9.
27. Linderborg K, et al. Potential mechanism for calvados-related oesophageal cancer. Food Chem Toxicol. 2008;46:476–9.
28. Secretan B, et al. A review of human carcinogens—part E: tobacco, areca nut, alcohol, coal smoke, and salted fish. Lancet Oncol. 2009;10:1033–4.
29. Slaughter DP, et al. Field cancerization in oral stratified squamous epithelium, clinical implications of multicentric origin. Cancer. 1953;6:963–8.
30. Mori M, et al. Lugol staining pattern and histology of esophageal lesions. Am J Gastroenterol. 1993;88:701–5.

31. Muto M, et al. Association of multiple Lugol-voiding lesions with synchronous and metachronous esophageal squamous cell carcinoma in patients with head and neck cancer. Gastrointest Endosc. 2002;56:517–21.
32. Katada C, et al. Alcohol consumption and multiple dysplastic lesions increase risk of squamous cell carcinoma in the esophagus, head, and neck. Gastroenterology. 2016;151:860–9.
33. Muto M, et al. Association between aldehyde dehydrogenase gene polymorphisms and the phenomenon of field cancerization in patients with head and neck cancer. Carcinogenesis. 2002;23:1759–65.
34. Yokoyama A, et al. Polymorphisms of alcohol dehydrogenase-1B and aldehyde dehydrogenase-2 and the blood and salivary ethanol and acetaldehyde concentrations of Japanese alcoholic men. Alcohol Clin Exp Res. 2010;34:1246–56.
35. Yokoyama A, et al. Salivary acetaldehyde concentration according to alcoholic beverage consumed and aldehyde dehydrogenase-2 genotype. Alcohol Clin Exp Res. 2008;32:1607–14.
36. Nieminen MT, et al. Local acetaldehyde: an essential role in alcohol-related upper gastrointestinal tract carcinogenesis. Cancers (Basel). 2018;10:pii: E11.
37. Dong YJ, et al. Expression and activities of class IV alcohol dehydrogenase and class III aldehyde dehydrogenase in human mouth. Alcohol. 1996;13:257–62.
38. Bik EM, et al. Bacterial diversity in the oral cavity of 10 healthy individuals. ISME J. 2010;4:962–74.
39. Kurkivuori J, et al. Acetaldehyde production from ethanol by oral streptococci. Oral Oncol. 2007;43:181–6.
40. Nieminen MT, et al. Acetaldehyde production from ethanol and glucose by non-*Candida albicans* yeasts in vitro. Oral Oncol. 2009;45:e245–8.
41. Uittamo J, et al. Chronic candidosis and oral cancer in APECED patients: production of carcinogenic acetaldehyde from glucose and ethanol by *Candida albicans*. Int J Cancer. 2009;124:754–6.
42. Vakevainen S, et al. High salivary acetaldehyde after a moderate dose of alcohol in ALDH2-deficient subjects: strong evidence for the local carcinogenic action of acetaldehyde. Alcohol Clin Exp Res. 2000;24:873–7.
43. Mizumoto A, et al. Molecular mechanisms of acetaldehyde-mediated carcinogenesis in squamous epithelium. Int J Mol Sci. 2017;18:E1943.
44. Wang M, et al. Identification of DNA adducts of acetaldehyde. Chem Res Toxicol. 2000;13:1149–57.
45. Fang JL, et al. Development of a ^{32}P-postlabelling method for the analysis of adducts arising through the reaction of acetaldehyde with 2′-deoxyguanosine-3′-monophosphate and DNA. Carcinogenesis. 1995;16:2177–85.
46. Hecht SS, et al. New DNA adducts of crotonaldehyde and acetaldehyde. Toxicology. 2001;166:31–6.
47. Matsuda T, et al. Increased formation of hepatic N2-ethylidene-2′-deoxyguanosine DNA adducts in aldehyde dehydrogenase 2-knockout mice treated with ethanol. Carcinogenesis. 2007;28:2363–6.
48. Balbo S, et al. Kinetics of DNA adduct formation in the oral cavity after drinking alcohol. Cancer Epidemiol Biomark Prev. 2012;21:601–8.
49. Balbo S, et al. N2-ethyldeoxyguanosine as a potential biomarker for assessing effects of alcohol consumption on DNA. Cancer Epidemiol Biomark Prev. 2008;17:3026–32.
50. Yukawa Y, et al. Combination of ADH1B*2/ALDH2*2 polymorphisms alters acetaldehyde-derived DNA damage in the blood of Japanese alcoholics. Cancer Sci. 2012;103:1651–5.
51. Balbo S, et al. Increased levels of the acetaldehyde-derived DNA adduct N2-ethyldeoxyguanosine in oral mucosa DNA from rhesus monkeys exposed to alcohol. Mutagenesis. 2016;31:553–8.
52. Amanuma Y, et al. Protective role of ALDH2 against acetaldehyde-derived DNA damage in oesophageal squamous epithelium. Sci Rep. 2015;5:14142.
53. Matsuda T, et al. Effective utilization of N2-ethyl-20-deoxyguanosine triphosphate during DNA synthesis catalyzed by mammalian replicative DNA polymerases. Biochemistry. 1999;38:929–35.

54. Upton DC, et al. Replication of N2-ethyldeoxyguanosine DNA adducts in the human embryonic kidney cell line 293. Chem Res Toxicol. 2006;19:960–7.
55. Garcia CC, et al. [13C2]-acetaldehyde promotes unequivocal formation of 1,N2-propano-2′-deoxyguanosine in human cells. J Am Chem Soc. 2011;133:9140–3.
56. Matsuda T, et al. Increased DNA damage in ALDH2-deficient alcoholics. Chem Res Toxicol. 2006;19:1374–8.
57. Mao H, et al. Duplex DNA catalyzes the chemical rearrangement of a malondialdehyde deoxyguanosine adduct. Proc Natl Acad Sci U S A. 1999;96:6615–20.
58. Minko IG, et al. Chemistry and biology of DNA containing 1,N2-deoxyguanosine adducts of the, unsaturated aldehydes acrolein, crotonaldehyde, and 4-hydroxynonenal. Chem Res Toxicol. 2009;22:759–78.
59. Brooks PJ, et al. DNA adducts from acetaldehyde: implications for alcohol-related carcinogenesis. Alcohol. 2005;35:187–93.
60. Matsuda T, et al. Specific tandem GG to TT base substitutions induced by acetaldehyde are due to intra-strand crosslinks between adjacent guanine bases. Nucleic Acids Res. 1998;26:1769–74.
61. Cho YJ, et al. Stereospecific formation of interstrand carbinolamine DNA cross-links by crotonaldehyde- and acetaldehyde-derived -CH3-OH-1,N2-propano-2′-deoxyguanosine adducts in the 50-CpG-30 sequence. Chem Res Toxicol. 2006;19:195–208.
62. Loureiro AP, et al. Trans,trans-2,4-decadienal-induced 1,N2-etheno-20-deoxyguanosine adduct formation. Chem Res Toxicol. 2000;13:601–9.
63. Tanaka K, et al. ALDH2 modulates autophagy flux to regulate acetaldehyde-mediated toxicity thresholds. Am J Cancer Res. 2016;6:781–96.
64. Akasaka S, et al. Mutagenicity of site-specifically located 1,N2-ethenoguanine in Chinese hamster ovary cell chromosomal DNA. Chem Res Toxicol. 1999;12:501–7.
65. Jansson T. The frequency of sister chromatid exchanges in human lymphocytes treated with ethanol and acetaldehyde. Hereditas. 1982;97:301–3.
66. Paget V, et al. Acetaldehyde-induced mutational pattern in the tumour suppressor gene tp53 analysed by use of a functional assay, the FASAY (functional analysis of separated alleles in yeast). Mutat Res. 2008;652:12–9.
67. Lin DC, et al. Genomic and molecular characterization of esophageal squamous cell carcinoma. Nat Genet. 2014;46:467–73.
68. Sawada G, et al. Genomic landscape of esophageal squamous cell carcinoma in a Japanese population. Gastroenterology. 2016;150:1171–82.
69. Cancer Genome Atlas Network. Comprehensive genomic characterization of head and neck squamous cell carcinomas. Nature. 2015;517:576–82.

Chapter 2
Gastroesophageal Reflux Diseases and Lifestyle Factors

Yasuhiro Fujiwara and Risa Uemura

Abstract Gastroesophageal reflux disease (GERD) is the most common upper gastrointestinal disorder and has been increasing in the past two decades in Japan. Several studies showed significant associations between GERD and lifestyle factors. In this chapter, we focused on obesity, metabolic syndrome, diabetes, hypertension, dyslipidemia, cigarette smoking, alcohol drinking, and late meals. We also discussed how these factors affect pathogenesis of GERD. We recommend modification of lifestyle factors associated with GERD as a basic therapeutic strategy.

Keywords GERD · Obesity · Metabolic syndrome · Smoking · Alcohol

2.1 Introduction

Gastroesophageal reflux disease (GERD) is the most common gastrointestinal (GI) disorder and the prevalence has been increasing in the past two decades in Japan (Fig. 2.1). Factors affecting the increased prevalence of GERD include a westernized lifestyle, an increase in gastric acid secretion in Japanese adults, a decrease in *Helicobacter pylori* infection, and changes in the concept of GERD, especially nonerosive reflux disease, defined as the presence of reflux symptoms without esophageal mucosal breaks on endoscopy [1, 2].

Several lifestyle factors such as obesity, cigarette smoking, alcohol drinking, exercise, excess eating, fatty or spicy foods, and late meals are commonly identified as risk factors for GERD [3]. Although proton-pump inhibitors (PPIs) are the first choice for treatment, the modification of lifestyle factors is advocated for GERD management because patients can choose therapeutic options by themselves. Systematic reviews have shown the benefits of lifestyle modifications on GERD and reflux symptoms, but there has been limited success in changing behaviors to reduce

Y. Fujiwara (✉) · R. Uemura
Department of Gastroenterology, Osaka City University Graduate School of Medicine, Osaka, Japan
e-mail: yasu@med.osaka-cu.ac.jp

H. Yoshiji, K. Kaji (eds.), *Alcoholic/Non-Alcoholic Digestive Diseases*,
https://doi.org/10.1007/978-981-13-1465-0_2

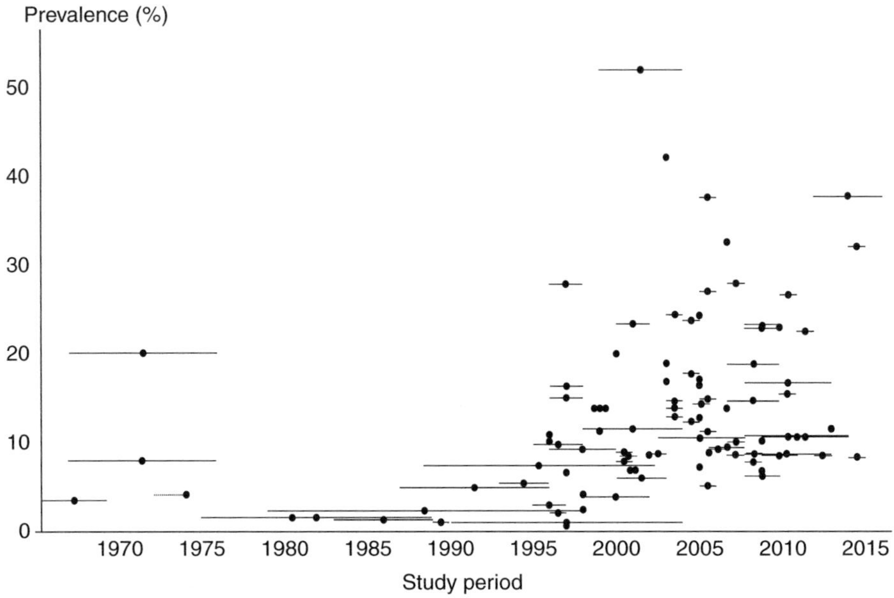

Fig. 2.1 Prevalence of GERD in the Japanese population. (modified from reference #1)

reflux symptoms [4]. However, a large Japanese study confirmed that lifestyle modification with PPI treatment significantly improved health-related quality of life (HR-QOL) in GERD patients compared with that using PPI treatment alone [5].

GERD has a multifactorial pathogenesis including lower esophageal sphincter (LES) dysfunction and impairment of esophageal clearance, but the most important factor is excess exposure to gastric acid in the esophageal lumen [3, 6–8]. In this chapter, we describe the associations between GERD and obesity, metabolic syndrome, cigarette smoking, alcohol drinking, and late meals. We also discussed how these lifestyle factors affect pathogenesis of GERD.

2.2 Obesity

Obesity is commonly defined by increased body mass index (BMI, >25 kg/m^2) and waist girth (males, >85 cm; females, >90 cm). Several studies reported that an increased BMI is associated with erosive GERD, and the odds ratio (OR) is approximately 1.5-fold for overweight (defined as BMI >25 kg/m^2), and two- to threefold for obese (defined as BMI >30 kg/m^2) individuals [9–11]. Western studies demonstrated that total obesity is associated with reflux symptoms, GERD, and esophageal adenocarcinoma. However, obesity as commonly found in Western countries is extremely rare in Japan. It is generally thought that intra-abdominal pressure in obese subjects contributes to abnormal esophageal acid exposure. Recently, several studies reported that not only simple obesity but also visceral fat obesity is associated with GERD [12, 13]. Waist girth is commonly used as a surrogate marker for visceral fat obesity. In fact, a large cross-sectional study of 80,110 individuals suggested that waist girth rather than BMI was associated with reflux symptoms [14].

As a mechanism, various cytokines including tumor necrosis factor (TNF)-α, interleukin (IL)-1, IL-6, and leptin are abnormally secreted by adipose tissue in visceral fat obesity. These cytokines may act systemically to influence and enhance inflammatory processes and affect both gastric secretion and LES function, since both IL-1β and TNFα stimulate gastrin release from human gastric antral fragments [15]. Baron analyzed data from four studies on maximum gastric acid output in healthy subjects and patients with peptic ulcer diseases, and found a significant positive correlation between body weight and gastric acid secretion [16]. Therefore, obesity is associated with GERD through enhancement of gastroesophageal reflux by an increase in intra-abdominal pressure, and increased gastric acid secretion and LES dysfunction caused by inflammatory cytokines.

Weight reduction plays an important role in GERD management [17]. Three randomized controlled trials in severely obese individuals compared weight reduction using gastric balloon distension with sham treatment combined with dietary guidance, physical exercise, and behavioral therapy, and showed reduced esophageal acid exposure with weight reduction [18–20]. Moreover, two large, prospective population-based cohort studies showed that weight reduction decreased reflux symptoms in a dose-dependent manner [21, 22]. Based on the pathophysiologic mechanisms, weight reduction in obese patients presumably will reduce the increased pressure on the gastroesophageal junction, thereby reducing reflux.

2.3 Metabolic Syndrome

Metabolic syndrome is defined as a cluster of metabolic abnormalities combined with visceral fat obesity, and is associated with cardiovascular diseases and other chronic disorders [23]. In Japan, metabolic syndrome is diagnosed using standard criteria including waist circumference beyond standard values and the presence of two or more of the following: (1) dyslipidemia, with low high-density lipoprotein cholesterol and/or elevated triglyceride, or medication for dyslipidemia; (2) impaired glucose tolerance, with elevated fasting plasma glucose, or medication for diabetes mellitus; and (3) hypertension, with elevated blood pressure, or medication for hypertension [24]. Moki et al. examined the association between erosive GERD and metabolic syndrome [25]. They found that male sex (odds ratio [OR] = 2.5), obesity (OR = 1.9), hyperglycemia (OR = 1.7), and hypertension (OR = 1.5) were independent risk factors for erosive GERD. Niigaki et al. also reported that metabolic syndrome is a reliable predictive factor for the prevalence of GERD, using data of 3775 persons who visited for routine health check-ups [26]. We describe the association between obesity or visceral fat obesity and GERD, and will discuss the association between GERD and each factor of metabolic syndrome in the following sections.

2.4 Diabetes Mellitus

Diabetic patients often complain of GI symptoms. Since diabetes mellitus and GERD share similar risk factors such as obesity, and since diabetes mellitus affects autonomic nerve function, a higher prevalence of GERD in diabetic patients is expected [27, 28]. Several studies showed that disease duration in diabetes [27, 28] and the presence of diabetic neuropathy [28] are associated with GERD. Since esophageal motility disorders and abnormal acid reflux in diabetic patients are associated with diabetic motor neuropathy [29], and since esophageal dysfunction is worsened with long disease duration [30], esophageal dysfunction may result in a higher prevalence of GERD in diabetic patients. There is another important issue concerning GERD in diabetic patients. Diabetic patients had fewer symptoms and sometimes patients have hematemesis without GERD symptoms [31].

2.5 Hypertension

Although a direct association between GERD and hypertension or blood pressure has not been reported, almost all physicians know that calcium antagonists are strongly related to GERD because calcium antagonists are listed in textbooks as potential drugs that impair LES function. Chow et al. reported that 20% of 15,662 patients treated with antihypertensive medications received acid-suppressive therapy [32]. Nitrates, calcium antagonists, and α1 antagonists were associated with increased OR for acid-suppressive therapy (OR 1.71 in nitrate users, OR 1.49 in calcium antagonist users, and OR 1.32 in α1 antagonist users). A change to a different antihypertensive medication might be considered when GERD patients with hypertension receive these drugs.

2.6 Dyslipidemia

Some studies showed that increased level of triglyceride and cholesterol were associated with GERD [33, 34], but there are several confounding factors between GERD and dyslipidemia. In addition, there is no study on the effect of medical treatment for dyslipidemia on GERD or reflux symptoms. Therefore, the association between GERD and hyperlipidemia remains unclear.

2.7 Cigarette Smoking

Watanabe et al. showed that current smoking was identified as a significant factor associated with GERD (OR = 1.35) [35]. Similarly, Nilsson et al. conducted a case control study of 3153 individuals with severe heartburn or regurgitation and 40,210 without reflux symptoms [36], and found a significant dose-response association between smoking and reflux symptoms.

If smoking is a significant risk factor for GERD, the question remains whether smoking cessation affects GERD and reflux symptoms. The HUNT study reported that quitting smoking improved reflux symptoms, but only in individuals of normal weight [37]. The HUNT study also reported risk factors for new onset of reflux symptoms [38]. The study showed that male sex and higher education were negatively associated with new-onset reflux symptoms, while an increase in BMI and previous or current smoking were positively associated, suggesting that smoking cessation was associated with new onset of reflux symptoms among patients with increased BMI upon smoking cessation. Our recent study showed that smoking cessation improved both GERD and HR-QOL [39]. We enrolled patients treated with varenicline, a nicotinic-receptor partial agonist, and surveyed reflux symptoms and HR-QOL before and 1 year after smoking cessation. A total of 141 patients achieved smoking cessation (success group) and 50 did not (failure group) at 1 year after treatment. The GERD improvement in the success group (43.9%) was significantly greater than that in the failure group (18.2%). The frequency of reflux symptoms only significantly decreased in the success group. There were no significant associations between new-onset GERD and clinical factors including increased BMI and successful smoking cessation. HR-QOL significantly improved only in the success group. Taken together, smoking is associated with GERD and smoking cessation improves GERD.

Early studies demonstrated that smoking reduced LES pressure and prolonged acid clearance through a decrease in saliva bicarbonate secretion. Kahrilas and Gupta showed that smokers exhibited lower LES pressures compared with nonsmokers, and smoking increased acid reflux events through an abrupt increase in intra-abdominal pressure during coughing or deep inspiration [40]. Two studies demonstrated that a short period (24 h) of abstaining from smoking did not influence esophageal acid exposure time in subjects both with and without reflux symptoms [41, 42]. However, Kadakia et al. showed a significant reduction in total acid reflux 48 h after smoking cessation [43].

2.8 Alcohol Drinking

Our epidemiological study using data of 4095 participants demonstrated that 276 (6.7%) were diagnosed as having GERD, and that moderate drinking (16–37 mL/day) and heavy drinking (≥38 mL/day) were associated with GERD [35]. Several studies reported the association between alcohol consumption and GERD [34, 36, 44, 45], but these results are conflicting. Unlike cigarette smoking, alcohol consumption is considered a triggering factor for GERD and reflux symptoms. Alcohol ingestion has been reported to reduce LES pressure and esophageal peristalsis, to increase acid exposure in the esophagus, and to have a direct noxious effect on the esophageal mucosa [46]. The effects of avoidance of alcohol drinking on GERD or reflux symptoms remain unclear, but avoidance is encouraged when alcohol consumption triggers reflux symptoms.

2.9 Late Meal

We examined 147 GERD patients and 294 age- and sex-matched controls without GERD symptoms and found that shorter dinner-to-bed time (<3 h) was significantly associated with GERD (OR = 7.45), compared with dinner-to-bed time 4 h or more [47]. In a crossover study, Piesman et al. assessed 32 GERD patients who were randomized to a high-fat meal either at 6 PM or 2 h before bedtime for two consecutive nights by using 48-h wireless pH monitoring [48]. Significantly more supine reflux was found to be associated with late meal consumption as compared with early meal consumption, especially in patients with hiatal hernia, overweight, and heartburn as their chief complaints. Late meals are related to enhanced postprandial reflux (within 2–3 h after a meal), which occurs during bedtime before and just after falling asleep, resulting in sleep disturbances. Therefore, avoidance of a late meal should be recommended in GERD patients, especially with those sleep disturbances.

2.10 Conclusions

Obesity including visceral fat obesity, metabolic syndrome, diabetes, hypertension, cigarette smoking, alcohol drinking, and late meals are associated with GERD through LES dysfunction, a decrease in esophageal clearance, increases in gastric acid secretion, and intra-abdominal pressure, or direct epithelial damage (Fig. 2.2). Lifestyle modification plays a crucial role in GERD treatment.

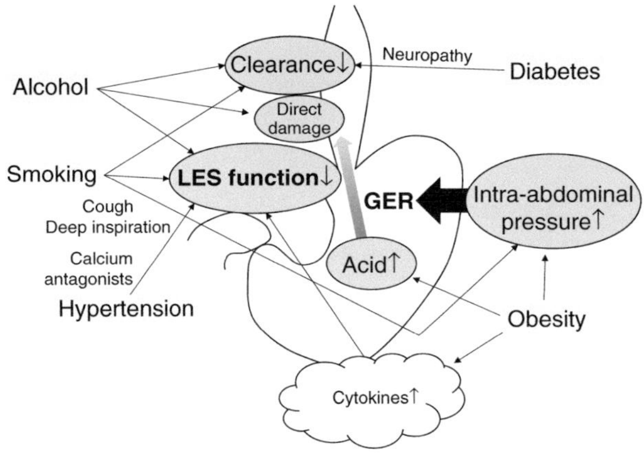

Fig. 2.2 Mechanisms of lifestyle factors in the pathogenesis of GERD. *LES* lower esophageal sphincter, *GER* gastroesophageal reflux

References

1. Fujiwara Y. Recent epidemiology of GERD in the Japanese population. Nihon Shokakibyo Gakkai Zasshi. 2017;114:1781–9.
2. Fujiwara Y, Arakawa T. Epidemiology and clinical characteristics of GERD in the Japanese population. J Gastroenterol. 2009;44:518–34.
3. Iwakiri K, Kinoshita Y, Habu Y, et al. Evidence-based clinical practice guidelines for gastroesophageal reflux disease 2015. J Gastroenterol. 2016;51:751–67.
4. Kaltenbach T, Crockett S, Gerson LB. Are lifestyle measures effective in patients with gastroesophageal reflux disease? An evidence-based approach. Arch Intern Med. 2006;166:965–71.
5. Kinoshita Y, Ashida K, Miwa H, et al. The impact of lifestyle modification on the health-related quality of life of patients with reflux esophagitis receiving treatment with a proton pump inhibitor. Am J Gastroenterol. 2009;104:1106–11.
6. El-Serag H. Role of obesity in GORD-related disorders. Gut. 2008;57:281–4.
7. El-Serag HB, Ergun GA, Pandolfino J, et al. Obesity increases oesophageal acid exposure. Gut. 2007;56:749–55.
8. Iwakiri K, Sugiura T, Hayashi Y, et al. Esophageal motility in Japanese patients with Barrett's esophagus. J Gastroenterol. 2003;38:1036–41.
9. El-Serag H. The association between obesity and GERD: a review of the epidemiological evidence. Dig Dis Sci. 2008;53:2307–12.
10. Corley DA, Kubo A. Body mass index and gastroesophageal reflux disease: a systematic review and meta-analysis. Am J Gastroenterol. 2006;101:2619–28.
11. Hampel H, Abraham NS, El-Serag HB. Meta-analysis: obesity and the risk for gastroesophageal reflux disease and its complications. Ann Intern Med. 2005;143:199–211.
12. Kang MS, Park DI, Oh SY, et al. Abdominal obesity is an independent risk factor for erosive esophagitis in a Korean population. J Gastroenterol Hepatol. 2007;22:1656–61.
13. Kato M, Watabe K, Hamasaki T, et al. Association of low serum adiponectin levels with erosive esophagitis in men: an analysis of 2405 subjects undergoing physical check-ups. J Gastroenterol. 2011;46:1361–7.
14. Corley DA, Kubo A, Zhao W. Abdominal obesity, ethnicity and gastro-oesophageal reflux symptoms. Gut. 2007;56:756–62.
15. Tilg H, Moschen AR. Visceral adipose tissue attacks beyond the liver: esophagogastric junction as a new target. Gastroenterology. 2010;139:1823–6.
16. Baron JH. Lean body mass, gastric acid, and peptic ulcer. Gut. 1969;10:637–42.
17. Ness-Jensen E, Hveem K, El-Serag H, et al. Lifestyle intervention in gastroesophageal reflux disease. Clin Gastroenterol Hepatol. 2016;14:175–82.e1–3.
18. Mathus-Vliegen LM, Tytgat GN. Twenty-four-hour pH measurements in morbid obesity: effects of massive overweight, weight loss and gastric distension. Eur J Gastroenterol Hepatol. 1996;8:635–40.
19. Mathus-Vliegen EM, Tygat GN. Gastro-oesophageal reflux in obese subjects: influence of overweight, weight loss and chronic gastric balloon distension. Scand J Gastroenterol. 2002;37:1246–52.
20. Mathus-Vliegen EM, van Weeren M, van Eerten PV. Los function and obesity: the impact of untreated obesity, weight loss, and chronic gastric balloon distension. Digestion. 2003;68:161–8.
21. Jacobson BC, Somers SC, Fuchs CS, et al. Body-mass index and symptoms of gastroesophageal reflux in women. N Engl J Med. 2006;354:2340–8.
22. Ness-Jensen E, Lindam A, Lagergren J, et al. Weight loss and reduction in gastroesophageal reflux. A prospective population-based cohort study: the HUNT study. Am J Gastroenterol. 2013;108:376–82.
23. Watanabe S, Hojo M, Nagahara A. Metabolic syndrome and gastrointestinal diseases. J Gastroenterol. 2007;42:267–74.

24. Sogabe M, Okahisa T, Kimura T, et al. Influence of metabolic syndrome on upper gastrointestinal disease. Clin J Gastroenterol. 2016;9:191–202.
25. Moki F, Kusano M, Mizuide M, et al. Association between reflux oesophagitis and features of the metabolic syndrome in Japan. Aliment Pharmacol Ther. 2007;26:1069–75.
26. Niigaki M, Adachi K, Hirakawa K, et al. Association between metabolic syndrome and prevalence of gastroesophageal reflux disease in a health screening facility in Japan. J Gastroenterol. 2013;48:463–72.
27. Nishida T, Tsuji S, Tsujii M, et al. Gastroesophageal reflux disease related to diabetes: analysis of 241 cases with type 2 diabetes mellitus. J Gastroenterol Hepatol. 2004;19:258–65.
28. Kase H, Hattori Y, Sato N, et al. Symptoms of gastroesophageal reflux in diabetes patients. Diabetes Res Clin Pract. 2008;79:e6–7.
29. Kinekawa F, Kubo F, Matsuda K, et al. Relationship between esophageal dysfunction and neuropathy in diabetic patients. Am J Gastroenterol. 2001;96:2026–32.
30. Kinekawa F, Kubo F, Matsuda K, et al. Esophageal function worsens with long duration of diabetes. J Gastroenterol. 2008;43:338–44.
31. Kinekawa F, Kubo F, Matsuda K, et al. Is the questionnaire for the assessment of gastroesophageal reflux useful for diabetic patients? Scand J Gastroenterol. 2005;40:1017–20.
32. Chow SL, Luzier AB, DiTusa L, et al. Acid-suppressive therapy use associated with antihypertensive agents. J Clin Pharmacol. 2001;41:750–6.
33. Park JH, Park DI, Kim HJ, et al. Metabolic syndrome is associated with erosive esophagitis. World J Gastroenterol. 2008;14:5442–7.
34. Matsuzaki J, Suzuki H, Kobayakawa M, et al. Association of visceral fat area, smoking, and alcohol consumption with reflux esophagitis and Barrett's esophagus in Japan. PLoS One. 2015;10:e0133865.
35. Watanabe Y, Fujiwara Y, Shiba M, et al. Cigarette smoking and alcohol consumption associated with gastro-oesophageal reflux disease in Japanese men. Scand J Gastroenterol. 2003;38:807–11.
36. Nilsson M, Johnsen R, Ye W, et al. Lifestyle related risk factors in the aetiology of gastro-oesophageal reflux. Gut. 2004;53:1730–5.
37. Ness-Jensen E, Lindam A, Lagergren J, et al. Tobacco smoking cessation and improved gastroesophageal reflux: a prospective population-based cohort study: the HUNT study. Am J Gastroenterol. 2014;109:171–7.
38. Hallan A, Bomme M, Hveem K, et al. Risk factors on the development of new-onset gastroesophageal reflux symptoms. A population-based prospective cohort study: the HUNT study. Am J Gastroenterol. 2015;110:393–400; quiz 401.
39. Kohata Y, Fujiwara Y, Watanabe T, et al. Long-term benefits of smoking cessation on gastroesophageal reflux disease and health-related quality of life. PLoS One. 2016;11:e0147860.
40. Kahrilas PJ, Gupta RR. Mechanisms of acid reflux associated with cigarette smoking. Gut. 1990;31:4–10.
41. Schindlbeck NE, Heinrich C, Dendorfer A, et al. Influence of smoking and esophageal intubation on esophageal pH-metry. Gastroenterology. 1987;92:1994–7.
42. Waring JP, Eastwood TF, Austin JM, et al. The immediate effects of cessation of cigarette smoking on gastroesophageal reflux. Am J Gastroenterol. 1989;84:1076–8.
43. Kadakia SC, Kikendall JW, Maydonovitch C, et al. Effect of cigarette smoking on gastroesophageal reflux measured by 24-h ambulatory esophageal pH monitoring. Am J Gastroenterol. 1995;90:1785–90.
44. Gunji T, Sato H, Iijima K, et al. Risk factors for erosive esophagitis: a cross-sectional study of a large number of Japanese males. J Gastroenterol. 2011;46:448–55.
45. Akiyama T, Inamori M, Iida H, et al. Alcohol consumption is associated with an increased risk of erosive esophagitis and Barrett's epithelium in Japanese men. BMC Gastroenterol. 2008;8:58.
46. Meining A, Classen M. The role of diet and lifestyle measures in the pathogenesis and treatment of gastroesophageal reflux disease. Am J Gastroenterol. 2000;95:2692–7.

47. Fujiwara Y, Machida A, Watanabe Y, et al. Association between dinner-to-bed time and gastroesophageal reflux disease. Am J Gastroenterol. 2005;100:2633–6.
48. Piesman M, Hwang I, Maydonovitch C, et al. Nocturnal reflux episodes following the administration of a standardized meal. Does timing matter? Am J Gastroenterol. 2007;102:2128–34.

Chapter 3
Post *Helicobacter pylori* Gastric Diseases

Kazunari Tominaga and Kazuhide Higuchi

Abstract A variety of researches have been focused on *Helicobacter pylori* (*H. pylori*) in gastroenterological field, and *H. pylori* has been recognized as etiologically responsible for gastritis-associated peptic ulcers and the majority of gastric cancers. The incidence rate of *H. pylori* infection is higher in Asian countries including Japan than in Western countries. However, past natural circumstances in Japan suitable for an inhabiting of *H. pylori* have been improved in parallel with the sanitary developments. In addition, the eradication therapy has been permitted with national insurance to most patients with *H. pylori* infection in 2013. As a result, the present infection rate is gradually decreasing. Based on the above surrounding environment, an age-depending decrease in acid secretion due to mucosal atrophy caused by chronic *H. pylori* infection is recently lacking. Therefore, certain acid secretion is continuously maintained with no age relationship. Accordingly, most Japanese physicians must switch their focus to the acid-related diseases (*H. pylori*-non-associated diseases) from the *H. pylori*-associated diseases throughout the entire generations.

As post *H. pylori* gastric diseases, this part will give the information about (1) *H. pylori*-negative mucosal injury excluding gastric cancer because it is introduced in the next chapter, (2) functional dyspepsia whose pathophysiology is in part associated with mucosal sensitivity to acid exposure, and (3) association of non-alcoholic fatty liver disease with gastroesophageal diseases.

Keywords Acid secretion · Chemical sensitivity · Functional disorders
Metabolic syndrome

K. Tominaga (✉)
Premier Developmental Research of Medicine, Osaka Medical College, Osaka, Japan

Second Department of Internal Medicine, Osaka Medical College, Osaka, Japan

K. Higuchi
Second Department of Internal Medicine, Osaka Medical College, Osaka, Japan

H. Yoshiji, K. Kaji (eds.), *Alcoholic/Non-Alcoholic Digestive Diseases*,
https://doi.org/10.1007/978-981-13-1465-0_3

3.1 *H. pylori*-Negative Mucosal Injury of the Stomach

3.1.1 H. pylori-*Negative Gastric Ulcer*

Since the discovery of *Helicobacter pylori* (*H. pylori*) in 1983, a variety of researches have been focused on the association of *H. pylori* with mucosal integrity and pathological disorders of the stomach [1–3]. Then, it has been proved that *H. pylori* infection makes abnormal circumstances of the stomach and causes various gastric diseases. In brief, *H. pylori* infection initially induces active acute gastritis, and sequentially chronic gastritis, atrophic gastritis, and intestinal metaplasia. All of these histological changes by chronic infection of *H. pylori* may lead to occurrence of peptic ulcers and gastric cancers (Fig. 3.1) [4]. Meanwhile, the World Health Organization classified *H. pylori* as a group I carcinogen in 1994 and confirmed that designation in 2012 [5, 6]. Therefore, it has been recognized that *H. pylori* is etiologically responsible for gastritis-associated peptic ulcers and the majority of gastric cancers as well as gastric mucosa-associated lymphoid tissue lymphoma (MALT lymphoma). In parallel with the above etiological evidences, various researches about the optimal regimens of *H. pylori* eradication have been gradually accumulated. In 2013, the eradication therapy was permitted to most *H. pylori*-positive patients with national insurance to treat the *H. pylori*-associated diseases such as peptic ulcers, MALT lymphoma, idiopathic thrombocytopenic purpura [7, 8] and prevent a recurrence of peptic ulcer and metachronous gastric cancer in Japan [9, 10]. As a result, the eradication therapy is widespread and often performed in various clinics. In addition, the Japanese natural circumstances suitable for inhabitation of *H. pylori* have been improved in parallel with the sanitary developments. In such trend of the times, the present infection rate of *H. pylori* was gradually lowered, although past infection rate was high in Japan. When considering the potent influences of *H. pylori* to the pathophysiology of the stomach, a simple question is firstly arising: Is there any *H. pylori*-negative gastric ulcer?

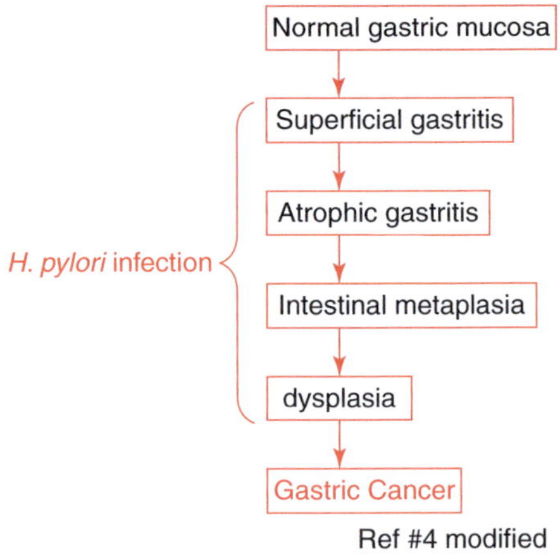

Fig. 3.1 General hypothesis of gastric carcinogenesis

The prevalence of peptic ulcer is indeed declining as well in various countries. A Japanese study reported that the prevalence rate of *pylori*-negative gastric ulcer was about 1.5–4.3%, whose etiology was mainly the use of non-steroidal anti-inflammatory drugs (NSAIDs) [11]. Another report revealed that the prevalence of idiopathic peptic ulcer (IPU) in patients with peptic ulcers is 12% in Japan [12]. Thus, certain proportion of *H. pylori*-negative gastric ulcers is present, although the true prevalence of IPUs not related to NSAIDs or *H pylori* infection is unknown.

Compared with those with simple *H. pylori*-positive ulcers, patients with IPUs were significantly older and more often had underlying comorbidities such as hypertension and hyperlipidemia. A presence of multiple underlying comorbidities significantly causes IPUs about four times higher compared to the patients without comorbidities. Furthermore, it is reported that patients with history of *H pylori*-negative idiopathic bleeding ulcer have a high risk of recurrent ulcer bleeding and mortality [13]. Therefore, in a post *H. pylori* era, it is important to consider underlying comorbidities such as lifestyle-related diseases including daily drug intake for evaluating the mechanism(s) of gastric mucosal injuries.

3.1.2 *Drug-Induced Gastric Ulcer (Recurrent Gastric Ulcer) After* H. pylori *Eradication*

As well as potent influences of *H. pylori*, it is well known that NSAIDs/low dose aspirin (LDA) causes gastric mucosal injury. The mechanism(s) is mediated via inhibition of cyclooxygenase and decrease in prostaglandin synthesis important for mucosal protection. Recently, the widespread use of complex anti-thrombotic therapy including LDA for lifestyle-related diseases such as cardiovascular diseases in the aging population has been recommended in various clinical fields. Therefore, it is expected that proportion of drug-induced (recurrent) gastric ulcers instead of peptic ulcers has been gradually increased and focused in a post *H. pylori* era. However, the detailed interaction between *H. pylori* infection (current or past) and NSAIDs use with the pathogenesis of peptic ulcers is still controversial [14, 15]. Interestingly, a meta-analysis indicated the interaction between NSAIDs use and *H. pylori* infection [16]. It is concluded that NSAIDs use is not associated with *H. pylori* infection in patients with peptic ulcer, whereas *H. pylori* eradication therapy reduces peptic ulcer incidence in NSAIDs users, especially in naive users and in the Asian population. Namely, *H. pylori* eradication therapy is useful for prevention of peptic ulcers in naive NSAIDs users, but the therapy may not be useful in continuous NSAIDs users (Fig. 3.2) [16]. However, these data cannot conclude whether NSAIDs-induced ulcers will increase in subjects without *H. pylori* infection in a post *H. pylori* era.

On the other hand, a recent interesting report showed that the long-term incidence of ulcer bleeding with LDA use is low after *H pylori* eradication alone despite a history of ulcer bleeding. Proton pump inhibitor (PPI) co-therapy can be used selectively in those *H pylori*-eradicated LDA users who require concomitant NSAIDs, anticoagulants, corticosteroids, or other antiplatelet drugs, while LDA

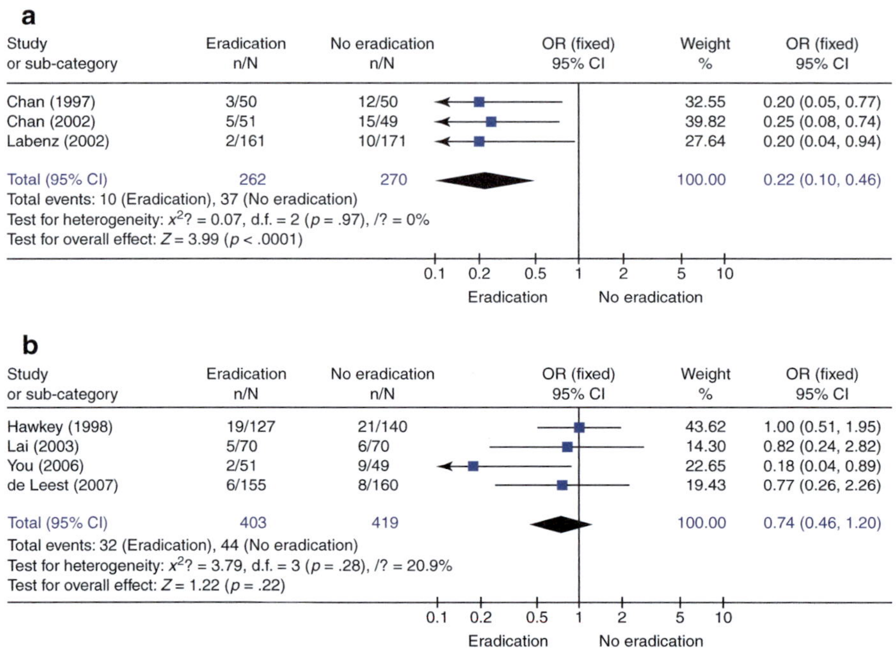

Fig. 3.2 Peptic ulcer and NSAIDs. (**a**) The incidence of peptic ulcer disease in non-steroidal anti-inflammatory drug (NSAID)-naive users with and those with no eradication therapy. (**b**) The incidence of peptic ulcer disease in chronic non-steroidal anti-inflammatory drug (NSAID) users with and those with no eradication therapy

users who developed ulcer bleeding without current or past *H pylori* infection are at high risk of recurrent bleeding and benefit most from PPI co-therapy [17]. These novel findings refined their treatment recommendations for LDA users who are at risk of ulcer bleeding.

The prevalence rate of peptic ulcer and ulcer bleeding in subjects without *H pylori* infection cannot be truly calculated even in a post *H pylori* era. However, the pathogenesis of gastric mucosal injuries caused by NSAIDs and LDA is proved to be similar. There is a recent background of upcoming increase in lifestyle-related diseases such as cardiovascular diseases and cerebral infarction. Therefore, an increased prevalence of drug-induced gastric ulcers may be easily inferred in parallel with an increased use of NSAIDs and LDA. Thus, Japanese medical doctors especially must understand an existence of *H. pylori*-negative gastric injuries, its pathogenesis, and therapeutic means.

3.2 Inflammation (Gastritis) and Acid Secretion

In a post *H pylori* era, how do the physiological functions of the stomach change after a withdrawal of potent influences of *H. pylori*? First, how about the prevalence of atrophic gastritis in Japan? There is an interesting retrospective report about this point investigating over a 40-year period [18]. In this report, for 1381 patients including 289 patients examined in the 1970s (158 men; mean age, 44.9 years), 787 in the 1990s (430 men; 44.2 years), and 305 in the 2010s (163 men; 53.2 years), severity of atrophy and *H. pylori* infection were investigated. Both the prevalence of atrophy in the antrum and corpus and the histological severity of atrophy and intestinal metaplasia were significantly lower in the 2010s compared to those in either the 1970s or 1990s [18]. Second, how about the secretion of gastric acid in Japan? There are population based studies in Japan. Both basal acid output (BAO) and maximal acid output (MAO) did not decrease with age in *H. pylori*-negative subjects, because gastric acid secretion decreased with progression of atrophic gastritis [19]. On the other hand, other report indicated that BAO and MAO gradually decreased with age in *H. pylori*-negative subjects [20, 21]. However, MAO in *H. pylori*-negative subjects has not changed over the past two decades (1990s and 2010s) in both non-elderly and elderly subjects. In etiology, prevalence rate of atrophic gastritis does not apparently decrease in gastroenterological field in Japan and an age-depending decrease in acid secretion due to gastric mucosal atrophy caused by chronic infection of *H. pylori* is lacking. This means that certain acid secretion is continuously maintained with no age relationship. In other words, the main attention in gastroenterology must be moved from the *H. pylori*-associated diseases to the acid-related diseases. Accordingly, most Japanese physicians must inevitably adapt to such changes throughout the entire generations.

3.3 Functional Dyspepsia Defined without *H. pylori* Infection: Hypersensitive Mucosa to Acid Exposure

By the way, in addition to understanding of the *H. pylori*-associated diseases, what are the acid-related gastric diseases? This must mean that acid sensitization is at least associated with the pathophysiology of the gastric diseases. A basic experimental study demonstrated that gastric acid is related to gastric chemonociception [22]. Direct acid exposure to the gastric mucosa is afferently transmitted to the brain via the capsaicin-sensitive sensory nerve and the vagal pathway but not spinal sensory pathways [22]. The HCl concentration-dependent (0.15 and 0.3 mol/L) excitation of medullary neurons is also in part associated with behavioral manifestations of pain [23]. In addition, histological inflammation of the stomach can be a trigger for hypersensitivity caused by acid exposure [23]. In human studies, exposure of gastric acid also induces various dyspeptic symptoms such as heavy feeling in the stomach, bloating, nausea or feeling sick, and belching [24]. The proportion of subjects developing symptoms by acid or water infusion was significantly greater in functional dyspepsia (FD) patients than healthy subjects, and particularly hypersensitivity to acid was observed in the FD patients [25]. Thus, hypersensitivity to gastric acid is one of the important mechanisms of the development of symptoms of FD which associates with multiple pathophysiological factors. As well as the previous meta-analysis (Fig. 3.3) [26], therapeutic efficacy for FD shown in recent individual studies using acid-suppressing agents such as H_2 receptor antagonists and PPIs can

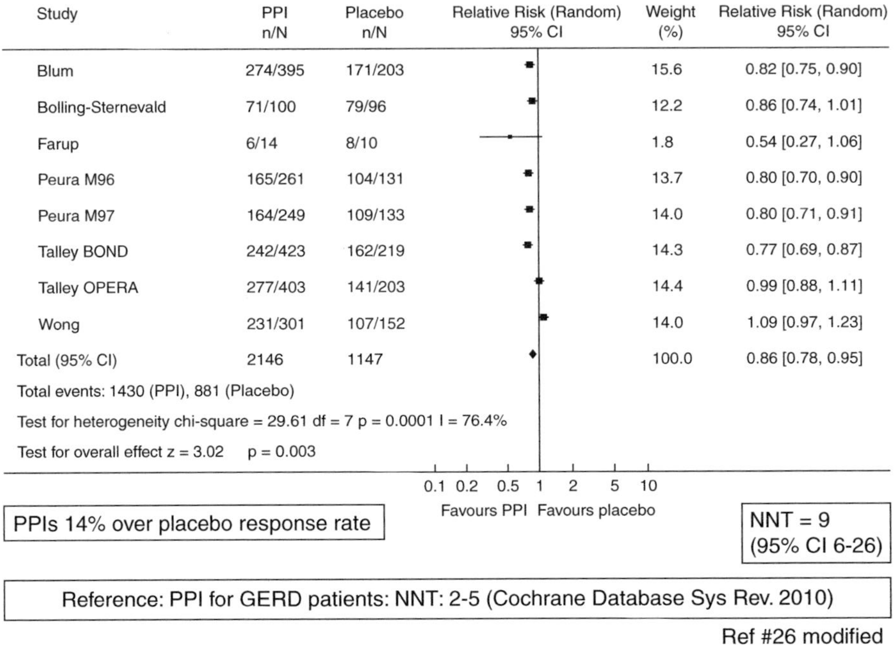

Fig. 3.3 Meta-analysis for double blinded randomized clinical trials using proton pump inhibitors for non-ulcer dyspepsia

be supportive for the above findings [27–30]. In addition, the Kyoto global consensus report has recently indicated that *H. pylori*-positive patients are differentially categorized using the diagnostic criteria of FD [31]. The Rome IV [32] and Japanese diagnostic criteria [33] also indicate that the true FD should be defined as *H. pylori*-negative status. Thus, among various gastric diseases in a post *H. pylori* era, FD may account the importance in the Japanese population with continuously maintained acid secretion.

3.4 Association of Non-alcoholic Fatty Liver Disease with Gastroesophageal Diseases

Prevalence rate of common diseases in gastroenterology has been changing in recent Japanese modern life. In such trend of the times, there is an increase in the rate of metabolic syndrome, a risk factor for lifestyle-related diseases in a post *H. pylori* era. For example, although gastric acid secretion has not increased over the past two decades in the Japanese population, the prevalence of gastroesophageal reflux diseases (GERD), a representative acid-related disease, has been increasing [17]. Such an etiological phenomenon may be partially due to an increased prevalence of metabolic syndrome including visceral obesity.

The pathogenesis of non-alcoholic fatty liver disease (NAFLD) closely relates to visceral obesity and insulin resistance. Insulin resistance is induced by imbalance of various humoral factors, e.g., adipokines [34]. Thus, NAFLD is thought as one of the hepatic manifestations of metabolic syndrome, because hyperglycemia, dyslipidemia, and hypertension are associated with NAFLD [35]. Considering common characteristic features of NAFLD and GERD such as visceral obesity, it is also suggested that GERD symptoms may be potentially present in patients with NAFLD, although patients with NAFLD do not generally complain of obvious abdominal symptoms. Meanwhile, we previously revealed a high prevalence (about 40%) of GERD symptoms in Japanese patients with NAFLD [36]. The risk factors associated with GERD symptoms were identified as serum triglyceride (TG) and total cholesterol levels (T-CHO) but not body mass index [36]. Intraduodenal administration of long chain TG after meal affects functions of lower esophageal sphincter such as contraction and relaxation [37, 38], and cholesterol of dietary nutrients enhances perception of the esophagus after intra-esophageal acid reflux [39]. In addition, serum TG levels are associated with non-erosive GERD [40] and erosive GERD [41] mediated via these mechanism(s). Thus, some reports support our previous findings. Therefore, an increase in serum TG and T-CHO levels as one of manifestations of hyperlipidemia mainly causes GERD symptoms but not common risk factor such as abdominal pressure caused by visceral obesity in patients with NAFLD (Fig. 3.4).

Hyperlipidemia is also closely related to obesity, and the concept of obesity-induced gastrointestinal neoplasia has been recognized. So, metabolic syndrome is a high risk for gastric cancer. Among various factors, as well as the microbiota and

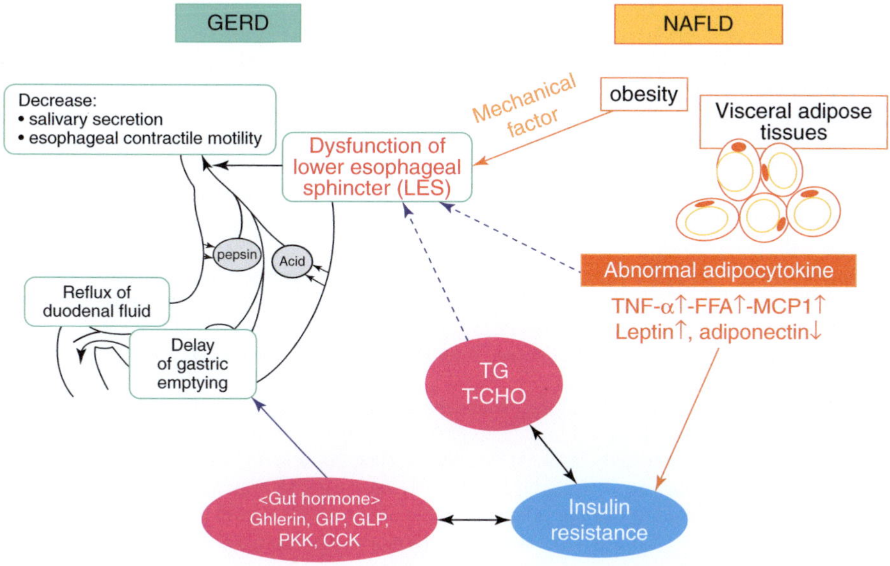

Fig. 3.4 Interaction of the pathogenesis between NAFLD and GERD

gastroesophageal reflux, high fat diet (HFD)-related malignancy is reported [42]. Recent experimental data showed that free fatty acids (FFAs) detected in the stomach of the HFD-fed mice impaired mitochondrial function and decreased the viability of parietal cells [43]. Furthermore, during HFD feeding (8–20 weeks), a total of 23% of the mice developed macroscopically distinct metaplastic lesions in the gastric corpus mucosa. Thus, dietary lipids induce parietal-cell damage and lead to the development of precancerous metaplasia. As a result, *H. pylori*-negative gastric cancer may be probably increased in future era of satiation.

3.5 Conclusions

In trend of the times as a post *H. pylori* era, it is easily expected that there appear some changes in prevalence rate of upper digestive tract diseases such as gastritis, gastric ulcers, and gastric cancers in Japan. Namely, apart from histological diseases of the stomach associated with *H. pylori* infection, symptom-based diseases or metabolism-related diseases without *H. pylori* infection may be progressively increased in the future. Hence, most of the Japanese physicians must correspond to such dramatic changes with a wide range of knowledge for both common gastric diseases due to the fact that the above old-fashioned diseases remain with certain probability even in the future.

References

1. Warren JR, Marshall BJ. Unidentified curved bacilli on gastric epithelium in active chronic gastritis. Lancet. 1983;1:1273–5.
2. Marshall BJ, Warren JR. Unidentified curved bacilli in the stomach of patients with gastritis and peptic ulceration. Lancet. 1984;1:1311–5.
3. Namekata T, Miki K, Kimmey M, Fritsche T, Hughes D, Moore D, et al. Chronic atrophic gastritis and *Helicobacter pylori* infection among Japanese Americans in Seattle. Am J Epidemiol. 2000;151:820–30.
4. Correa P. Human gastric carcinogenesis: a multistep and multifactorial process--First American Cancer Society Award Lecture on Cancer Epidemiology and Prevention. Cancer Res. 1992;52:6735–40.
5. International Agency for Research on Cancer, World Health Organization. Schistosomes, liver flukes and *Helicobacter pylori*. IARC Monogr Eval Carcinog Risks Hum. 1994;61:177–241.
6. International Agency for Research on Cancer. *Helicobacter pylori*. Biologic agents: a review of human carcinogens, vol. 100B. Leon: International Agency for Research on Cancer; 2012. p. 385–435.
7. Higuchi K, Fujiwara Y, Tominaga K, Watanabe T, Shiba M, Nakamura S, et al. Is eradication sufficient to heal gastric ulcers in patients infected with *Helicobacter pylori*? A randomized, controlled, prospective study. Aliment Pharmacol Ther. 2003;17:111–7.
8. Tsumoto C, Tominaga K, Okazaki H, Tanigawa T, Yamagami H, Watanabe K, et al. Long-term efficacy of *Helicobacter pylori* eradication in patients with idiopathic thrombocytopenic purpura: 7-year follow-up prospective study. Ann Hematol. 2009;88:789–93.

9. Miwa H, Sakaki N, Sugano K, Sekine H, Higuchi K, Uemura N, et al. Recurrent peptic ulcers in patients following successful *Helicobacter pylori* eradication: a multicenter study of 4940 patients. Helicobacter. 2004;9:9–16.
10. Fukase K, Kato M, Kikuchi S, Inoue K, Uemura N, Okamoto S, et al. Effect of eradication of *Helicobacter pylori* on incidence of metachronous gastric carcinoma after endoscopic resection of early gastric cancer: an open-label, randomised controlled trial. Lancet. 2008;372:392–7.
11. Aoyama N, Shinoda Y, Matsushima Y, Shirasaka D, Kinoshita Y, Kasuga M, et al. Helicobacter pylori-negative peptic ulcer in Japan: which contributes most to peptic ulcer development, *Helicobacter pylori*, NSAIDS or stress? J Gastroenterol. 2000;35(Suppl 12):33–7.
12. Kanno T, Iijima K, Abe Y, Yagi M, Asonuma S, Ohyauchi M, et al. A multicenter prospective study on the prevalence of *Helicobacter pylori*-negative and nonsteroidal anti-inflammatory drugs-negative idiopathic peptic ulcers in Japan. J Gastroenterol Hepatol. 2015;30:842–8.
13. Wong GL, Wong VW, Chan Y, Ching JY, Au K, Hui AJ, et al. High incidence of mortality and recurrent bleeding in patients with *Helicobacter pylori*-negative idiopathic bleeding ulcers. Gastroenterology. 2009;137:525–31.
14. Hawkey CJ, Tulassay Z, Szczepanski L, van Rensburg CJ, Filipowicz-Sosnowska A, Lanas A, et al. Randomised controlled trial of *Helicobacter pylori* eradication in patients on non-steroidal anti-inflammatory drugs: HELP NSAIDs study. Helicobacter eradication for lesion prevention. Lancet. 1998;352:1016–21.
15. de Leest HT, Steen KS, Lems WF, Bijlsma JW, van de Laar MA, Huisman AM, et al. Eradication of *Helicobacter pylori* does not reduce the incidence of gastroduodenal ulcers in patients on long-term NSAID treatment: double-blind, randomized, placebo-controlled trial. Helicobacter. 2007;12:477–85.
16. Tang CL, Ye F, Liu W, Pan XL, Qian J, Zhang GX. Eradication of *Helicobacter pylori* infection reduces the incidence of peptic ulcer disease in patients using nonsteroidal anti-inflammatory drugs: a meta-analysis. Helicobacter. 2012;17:286–96.
17. Chan FK, Ching JY, Suen BY, Tse YK, Wu JC, Sung JJ. Effects of *Helicobacter pylori* infection on long-term risk of peptic ulcer bleeding in low-dose aspirin users. Gastroenterology. 2013;144:528–35.
18. Kamada T, Haruma K, Ito M, Inoue K, Manabe N, Matsumoto H, et al. Time trends in *Helicobacter pylori* infection and atrophic gastritis over 40 years in Japan. Helicobacter. 2015;20:192–8.
19. Haruma K, Kamada T, Kawaguchi H, Okamoto S, Yoshihara M, Sumii K, et al. Effect of age and *Helicobacter pylori* infection on gastric acid secretion. J Gastroenterol Hepatol. 2000;15:277–83.
20. Kinoshita Y, Kawanami C, Kishi K, Nakata H, Seino Y, Chiba T. *Helicobacter pylori* independent chronological change in gastric acid secretion in the Japanese. Gut. 1997;41:452–8.
21. Ishimura N, Owada Y, Aimi M, Oshima T, Kamada T, Inoue K, et al. No increase in gastric acid secretion in healthy Japanese over the past two decades. J Gastroenterol. 2015;50:844–52.
22. Schuligoi R, Joci M, Heinemann A, Scho¨ninkle E, Pabst MA, Holzer P. Gastric acid–evoked c-fos messenger RNA expression in rat brainstem is signaled by capsaicin-resistant vagal afferents. Gastroenterology. 1998;115:649–60.
23. Lamb K, Kang YM, Gebhart GF, Bielefeldt K. Gastric inflammation triggers hypersensitivity to acid in awake rats. Gastroenterology. 2003;125:1410–8.
24. Miwa H, Nakajima K, Yamaguchi K, Fujimoto K, Veldhuyzen VAN Zanten SJ, et al. Generation of dyspeptic symptoms by direct acid infusion into the stomach of healthy Japanese subjects. Aliment Pharmacol Ther. 2007;26:257–64.
25. Oshima T, Okugawa T, Tomita T, Sakurai J, Toyoshima F, Watari J, et al. Generation of dyspeptic symptoms by direct acid and water infusion into the stomachs of functional dyspepsia patients and healthy subjects. Aliment Pharmacol Ther. 2012:175:175–82.
26. Moayyedi P, Soo S, Deeks J, Delaney B, Innes M, Forman D. Pharmacological interventions for non-ulcer dyspepsia. Cochrane Database Syst Rev. 2006;(5):178–85.

27. Peura DA, Kovacs TO, Metz DC, Siepman N, Pilmer BL, Talley NJ. Lansoprazole in the treatment of functional dyspepsia: two double-blind, randomized, placebo-controlled trials. Am J Med. 2004;116:740–8.
28. van Zanten SV, Armstrong D, Chiba N, Flook N, White RJ, Chakraborty B, et al. Esomeprazole 40 mg once a day in patients with functional dyspepsia: the randomized, placebo-controlled "ENTER" trial. Am J Gastroenterol. 2006;101:2096–106.
29. Iwakiri R, Tominaga K, Furuta K, Inamori M, Furuta T, Masuyama H, et al. Randomised clinical trial: rabeprazole improves symptoms in patients with functional dyspepsia in Japan. Aliment Pharmacol Ther. 2013;38:729–40.
30. Sakurai K, Nagahara A, Inoue K, Akiyama J, Mabe K, Suzuki J, et al. Efficacy of omeprazole, famotidine, mosapride and teprenone in patients with upper gastrointestinal symptoms: an omeprazole-controlled randomized study (J-FOCUS). BMC Gastroenterol. 2012;12:42. https://doi.org/10.1186/1471-230X-12-42.
31. Sugano K, Tack J, Kuipers EJ, Graham DY, El-Omar EM, Miura S, et al. Kyoto global consensus report on *Helicobacter pylori* gastritis. Gut. 2015;64:1353–67.
32. Stanghellini V, Chan FK, Hasler WL, Malagelada JR, Suzuki H, Tack J, et al. Gastroduodenal Disorders. Gastroenterology. 2016;150:1380–92.
33. Miwa H, Kusano M, Arisawa T, Oshima T, Kato M, Joh T, et al. Evidence-based clinical practice guidelines for functional dyspepsia. J Gastroenterol. 2015;50:125–39.
34. Xu H, Barnes GT, Yang Q, Tan G, Yang D, Chou CJ, et al. Chronic inflammation in fat plays a crucial role in the development of obesity-related insulin resistance. J Clin Invest. 2003;112:1821–30.
35. Marchesini G, Bugianesi E, Forlani G, Cerrelli F, Lenzi M, Manini R, et al. Nonalcoholic fatty liver, steatohepatitis, and the metabolic syndrome. Hepatology. 2003;37:917–23.
36. Fujikawa Y, Tominaga K, Fujii H, Machida H, Okazaki H, Yamagami H, et al. High prevalence of gastroesophageal reflux symptoms in patients with non-alcoholic fatty liver disease associated with serum levels of triglyceride and cholesterol but not simple visceral obesity. Digestion. 2012;86:228–37.
37. Ledeboer M, Mascle AAM, Biemond I, Lamers CBHW. Effect of medium- and long-chain triglycerides onlower esophageal sphincter pressure: role of CCK. Am J Phys. 1998;274:1160–5.
38. Trudgill NJ, Riley SA. Tansient lower esophageal sphincter relaxations are no more frequent in patients with gastroesophageal reflux disease than in asymptomatic volunteers. Am J Gastroenterol. 2001;96:2569–74.
39. Shapiro M, Green C, Bautista M, Dekel R, Risner-Adler S, Whitacre R, et al. Assessment of dietary nutrients that influence perception of intra-oesophageal acid reflux events in patients with gastro-oesophageal reflux disease. Aliment Pharmacol Ther. 2007;25:93–101.
40. Matsuzaki J, Suzuki H, Iwasaki E, Yokoyama H, Sugino Y, Hibi T. Serum lipid levels are positively associated with non-erosive reflux disease, but not with functional heartburn. Neurogastroenterol Motil. 2010;22:965–70.
41. Wu P, Ma L, Dai GX, Chen Y, Tong YL, Wang C, et al. The association of metabolic syndrome with reflux esophagitis: a case-control study. Neurogastroenterol Motil. 2011;23:989–94.
42. Schulz MD, Atay C, Heringer J, Romrig FK, Schwitalla S, Aydin B, et al. High-fat-diet-mediated dysbiosis promotes intestinal carcinogenesis independently of obesity. Nature. 2014;514:508–12.
43. Hirata Y, Sezaki T, Tamura-Nakano M, Oyama C, Hagiwara T, Ishikawa T, et al. Fatty acids in a high-fat diet potentially induce gastric parietal-cell damage and metaplasia in mice. J Gastroenterol. 2017;52:889–903.

Chapter 4
New Perspectives in Gastric Cancer: *Helicobacter pylori*-Uninfected Pure Signet Ring Cell Carcinoma

Takeshi Setoyama, Shin'ichi Miyamoto, Mitsuhiro Nikaido, and Hiroshi Seno

Abstract Although gastric cancer incidence and mortality rates remain high in Japan, they have decreased in recent years. This decline is thought to be attributable to the reduction of *Helicobacter pylori* (HP) infection rate (approximately 50% of the population born in the 1940s vs. 10% in the 1980s). However, some studies on HP-uninfected gastric cancer have reported that the prevalence of this type of cancer accounted for 5% at most. HP-uninfected gastric cancers include lesions related to autoimmune gastritis, Epstein–Barr virus infection, genetic factors such as hereditary diffuse gastric cancer (HDGC), and sporadic/nonhereditary cancers. Among sporadic HP-uninfected gastric cancers, pure signet ring cell carcinomas are reported to be the most common. In this chapter, clinicopathological characteristics of this type of cancer are discussed, compared with a case of HDGC. And speculation about the carcinogenic mechanisms (mainly focusing on *CDH1* gene alteration) based on the evidences obtained from previous excellent mouse models are also introduced here.

Keywords *Helicobacter pylori*-uninfected gastric cancer · Signet ring cell carcinoma · E-cadherin · *CDH1* gene alteration

4.1 Introduction

Gastric cancer is the third leading cause of cancer deaths worldwide, accounting for 723,100 deaths annually and an estimated 951,600 new cases in 2012 [1]. *Helicobacter pylori* (HP) infection is the most important etiologic factor for chronic

T. Setoyama
Department of Gastroenterology and Hepatology, Osaka Red Cross Hospital, Osaka, Japan
e-mail: takeseto@kuhp.kyoto-u.ac.jp

S. Miyamoto (✉) · M. Nikaido · H. Seno
Department of Gastroenterology and Hepatology, Kyoto University Graduate School of Medicine, Kyoto, Japan
e-mail: shmiyamo@kuhp.kyoto-u.ac.jp; seno@kuhp.kyoto-u.ac.jp

H. Yoshiji, K. Kaji (eds.), *Alcoholic/Non-Alcoholic Digestive Diseases*,
https://doi.org/10.1007/978-981-13-1465-0_4

gastritis and gastric cancer, and 89% of non-cardiac gastric cancers are known to be attributable to HP infection [2, 3]. Recently, it has been demonstrated in many reports that the eradication of HP is associated with a significantly lower risk of gastric cancer (pooled incidence rate ratio about 0.50) [4, 5].

Although gastric cancer incidence and mortality rates remain high in Japan, they have decreased in recent years [1, 6]. This recent decline is thought to be attributable to the reduction of HP infection rate caused by improvement of sanitary conditions and widespread application of eradication therapy [2, 3, 7]. However, some studies on HP-negative gastric cancer have reported that the prevalence of this type of cancer ranges from 0.42% to 5.4% [8, 9]. The frequency of HP-negative gastric cancer may relatively increase, even though the prevalence of all gastric cancers has decreased owing to the decline in HP infection. HP-negative gastric cancers include lesions related to autoimmune gastritis (AIG), Epstein–Barr virus (EBV) infection, genetic factors such as hereditary diffuse gastric cancer (HDGC), and sporadic/nonhereditary cancers [9–11].

AIG is an autoimmune disease with a prevalence of about 2% in the general population. It is a chronic inflammatory gastric disease that is limited to the fundus and body of the stomach, and is most commonly associated with pernicious anemia. Autoantibodies to the gastric parietal cells directed against the gastric H^+/K^+-ATPase and intrinsic factor are commonly described in these patients, who have a threefold increased risk of gastric carcinomas, and the annual incidence of gastric cancer ranges from 0.1% to 1.0% [12–14].

EBV-positive gastric cancer was defined as one of four molecular tumor classification subgroups by The Cancer Genome Atlas Research Network, and EBV is found within malignant epithelial cells in 9% of gastric cancers [15]. Most of these cancers are located in the fundus or the body of the stomach, and tumors positive for EBV are mostly found in men (81%) [11, 15, 16].

Truly hereditary cases are thought to account for 1–3% of all gastric cancers and consist of three main syndromes: HDGC, gastric adenocarcinoma and proximal polyposis of the stomach, and familial intestinal gastric cancer. A genetic basis, a causative mutation in *CDH1*, has been found in only about 40% of HDGC cases [10, 11, 17, 18]. A recent study on HDGC reported that by the age of 80 years, the cumulative incidence of gastric cancer is 70% for men and 56% for women [18].

Among sporadic HP-uninfected gastric cancers, relatively small pure (without a component of poorly differentiated carcinoma) signet ring cell carcinomas (SRCCs) are reported to be the most common. However, the carcinogenic mechanisms of this carcinoma are not clear [9, 19–21].

4.2 Diagnostic Criteria for HP-Uninfected Gastric Cancer

The reported prevalence of HP-negative gastric cancer varies because many different types of tests are routinely used to diagnose HP infection, and the diagnostic criteria for "HP-negative" are not yet established. This variation can be explained in part by the fact that cases with past infection were included in some reports. Excluding cases in individuals with past HP infection, the prevalence of "HP-uninfected" gastric cancer is calculated as 0.42–2.3% [8, 9, 21, 22]. With reference to those previous reports, in our institution, "HP-uninfected" is defined if the person meets all five of the following criteria: [1] no history of HP eradication [2], negative urea breath test [3], blood HP antigen level <3 U/mL [4], histologically confirmed HP negative, and [5] no endoscopic findings of mucosal atrophy.

4.3 Characteristics of HP-Uninfected Intramucosal Pure Signet Ring Cell Carcinoma

4.3.1 Case Presentation of HDGC

A 26-year-old woman visited our hospital for a detailed examination for gastric cancer because her older brother had died at a young age from advanced gastric cancer with the *CDH1* germline mutation (nonsense mutation at exon 3, unpublished data). Esophagogastroduodenoscopy showed a 25-mm, discolored, flat lesion located on the greater curvature of the middle gastric body. Because the histopathology of a biopsy specimen revealed SRCC, this family was diagnosed with HDGC according to the consensus guidelines [10, 23]. The patient carried the same *CDH1* germline mutation as her older brother. She underwent total gastrectomy, and three small intramucosal SRCCs were confirmed. Interestingly, this lesion met our criteria for HP-uninfected gastric cancer.

4.3.2 HP-Uninfected Pure Signet Ring Cell Carcinoma

Including this HDGC case (case 1), eight cases of HP-uninfected SRCC have been diagnosed in our institution from October 2014 to December 2017; the other seven cases were sporadic (Table 4.1). The mean age of the patients was 53 years, and six of the eight patients were men. These patients' characteristics were similar to those in a previous report [19]. These cancers had characteristic endoscopy findings that showed discolored and flat lesions measuring 15 mm or less in the middle body of the stomach, especially around the borderline zone of the gastric gland [9]. Furthermore, in all cases, histopathology revealed pure intramucosal SRCC spreading in the proliferative zone. A representative case (case 5) is shown in Fig. 4.1 (endoscopic findings) and Fig. 4.2 (hematoxylin and eosin staining). A previous study showed that the MIB-1 labeling index (an indicator of the proliferation capacity) was significantly lower in the HP-uninfected SRCC than in HP-positive cases [19]. This suggested that HP-uninfected SRCC might be confined to the lamina propria, resulting in slow progression and a better prognosis. In fact, among our cases, case 2 was diagnosed with a 3-mm intramucosal SRCC that showed no notable change endoscopically for over a year. Furthermore, all cases were negative for lymphovascular invasion.

Table 4.1 Clinicopathological characteristics of HP-uninfected pure signet ring cell carcinoma

	Age	Gender	Location	Histology	Size (mm)	Solitary or multiple	Depth of invasion	ly	v	Treatment	History of cancer
Case 1	28	F	M + L	Pure SRCC	25/10/2	Multiple (three lesions)	Intramucosal	–	–	Total gastrectomy	None
Case 2	48	M	M	Pure SRCC	3	Solitary	Intramucosal	–	–	Endoscopic resection	None
Case 3	61	M	M	Pure SRCC	13	Solitary	Intramucosal	–	–	Endoscopic resection	None
Case 4	63	M	M	Pure SRCC	14	Solitary	Intramucosal	–	–	Endoscopic resection	Esophageal cancer Pharyngel cancer
Case 5	56	F	M	Pure SRCC	10	Solitary	Intramucosal	–	–	Endoscopic resection	None
Case 6	73	M	M	Pure SRCC	7	Solitary	Intramucosal	–	–	Endoscopic resection	Hepatocellular carcinoma
Case 7	50	M	M	Pure SRCC	12	Solitary	Intramucosal	–	–	Endoscopic resection	None
Case 8	40	M	M	Pure SRCC	6	Solitary	Intramucosal	–	–	Endoscopic resection	None

M middle gastric body, *L* lower gastric body, *SRCC* signet ring cell carcinoma, *ly* lymphatic invasion, *v* venous invasion

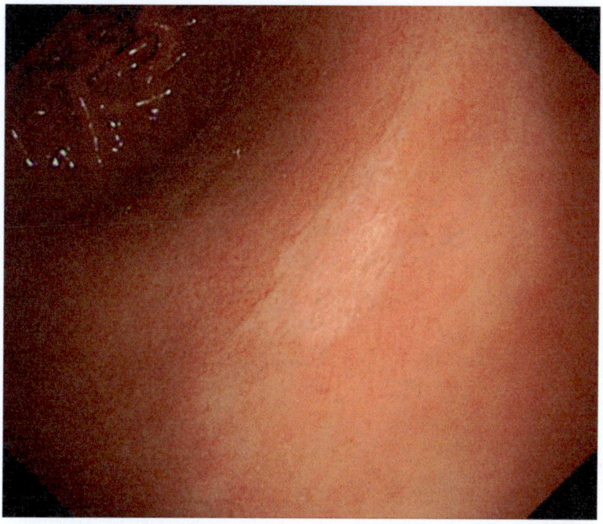

Fig. 4.1 Typical endoscopic findings of *Helicobacter pylori*-uninfected intramucosal pure signet ring cell carcinoma. A discolored and flat lesion, 10-mm in diameter, is located at the posterior wall of the middle gastric body

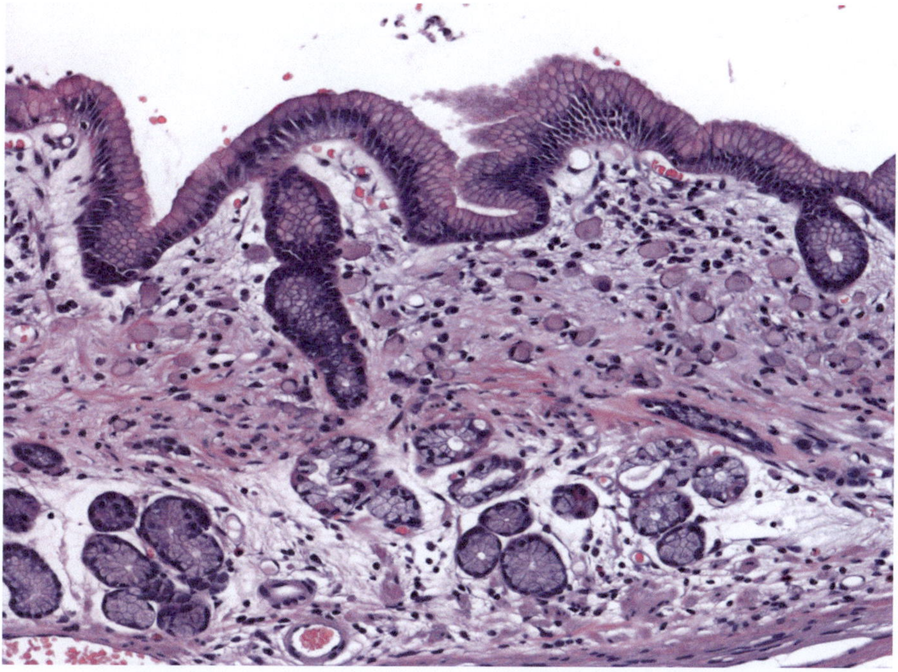

Fig. 4.2 Typical pathological growth pattern of *Helicobacter pylori*-uninfected intramucosal pure signet ring cell carcinoma. Pathological findings (hematoxylin and eosin staining, 20-fold magnification) revealed cancer cells extending transversally in the proliferative zone that were not exposed to the gastric mucosal surface

4.4 Speculation about the Carcinogenic Mechanisms of HP-Uninfected Pure Signet Ring Cell Carcinoma

A previous study reported that in prophylactic gastrectomy specimens obtained from carriers of the germline *CDH1* mutation, the neoplastic cells displayed a pure signet ring cell phenotype, and carcinoma was confined to the mucosa with the majority of foci occupying the upper half of the mucosa [24]. These characteristic patterns of growth [19, 21] and pattern of immunohistochemical staining for E-cadherin are also similar to those seen in the sporadic intramucosal HP-uninfected SRCC (Fig. 4.3).

CDH1 "germline" alteration is well-known as a causative mechanism of HDGC, although "somatic" *CDH1* alterations have been found in sporadic diffuse-type gastric cancers [25–27].

Humar et al. reported that untreated *Cdh1*$^{+/-}$ mice had only a low incidence of murine SRCC (5%); however, N-methyl-N-nitrosourea (MNU)-treated *Cdh1*$^{+/-}$ mice developed murine SRCC at 11 times the incidence of either untreated *Cdh1*$^{+/-}$ mice or MNU-treated wild-type mice [28]. Mimata et al. also reported that in

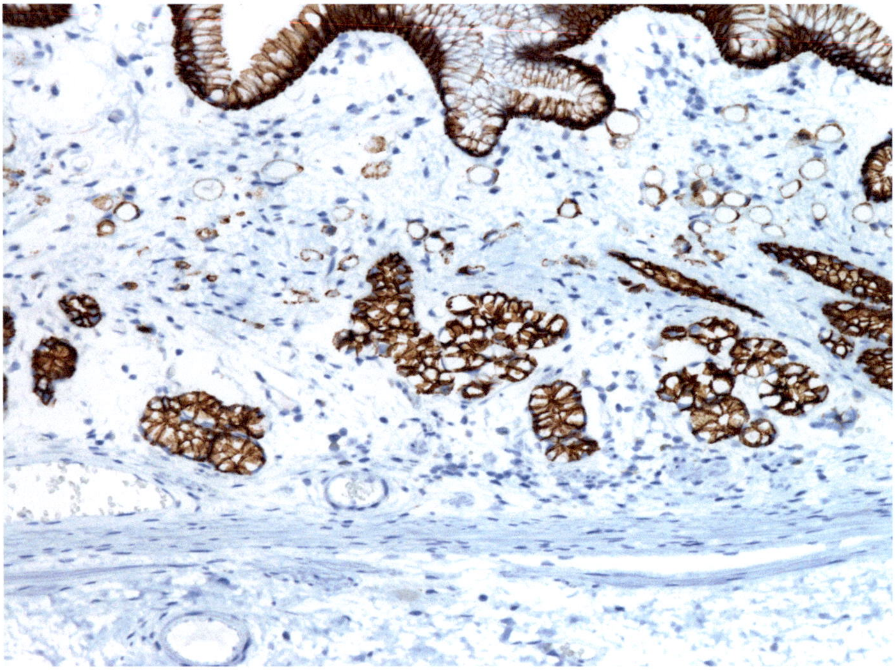

Fig. 4.3 Pattern of immunohistochemical staining for E-cadherin in *Helicobacter pylori*-uninfected intramucosal pure signet ring cell carcinoma. Immunohistochemistry (20-fold magnification) revealed weak E-cadherin expression on cancer cells compared with the normal crypt epithelium and fundic gland

parietal cell-specific *Cdh1* knockout mice, signet ring-like cells morphologically similar to human SRCC were found in clusters, although invasive gastric carcinoma was not induced [29].

A recent study [30] showed that knocking out the *Cdh1* gene in Mist1-expressing cells (quiescent stem cells in the gastric gland) in mice resulted in the development of atypical cell foci, consistent with early signet ring cell morphology, which recapitulated the earliest events in the pathogenesis of human SRCC. However, the number of these atypical cells gradually declined until finally disappearing, which suggested again that E-cadherin loss alone is insufficient to maintain SRCC. In the same mice with chronic inflammation induced by *Helicobacter felis* (HF) infection, these atypical cell foci were preserved and expanded. Furthermore, administration of dexamethasone to these HF-infected mice reduced the number of signet ring cell foci to the same level as in uninfected control mice.

These results suggested that the loss of E-cadherin function alone is not sufficient for invasive cancer formation, and that synergistic effects of inactivated *CDH1* and other oncogenic factors are necessary for the development of invasive diffuse (not pure SRCC) gastric cancer.

In another study of early cancer, human intestinal-type gastric cancer showed a much higher frequency of *TP53* mutations than did diffuse-type gastric cancer, and when early and advanced diffuse-type tumors were compared, a significant increase was observed in the advanced tumors [31]. These results suggested that *TP53* alterations could be mainly associated with tumor progression in diffuse-type cancer. In fact, Shimada et al. [32] reported that invasive cancers composed of signet ring cells and poorly differentiated carcinoma cells very histologically similar to human diffuse gastric cancer were observed in parietal cell-specific *Cdh1* and *Trp53* double-knockout mice. After 12 months, these cancer cells metastasized to the lymph nodes (about 40%), but not the distant organs, in an immunodeficient mouse. Hayakawa et al also demonstrated that the addition of *Trp53* mutation in their setting led to invasive diffuse gastric cancer within 9 months [30].

4.5 Future Directions

The prevalence of HP-uninfected gastric cancer is still low and is thought to represent approximately 1% of all gastric cancers in Japan. Among these, the opportunity to encounter intramucosal pure SRCC may gradually increase.

Excellent mouse models have suggested that HP-uninfected intramucosal pure SRCC could develop as a result of the loss of E-cadherin function alone, but that it could not persist without additional factors such as chronic inflammation leading to *Trp53* mutations. Because HP-uninfected intramucosal pure SRCC cases are rare, genetic analysis has not yet been performed. Further studies are needed to elucidate the detailed carcinogenic mechanism and biological behavior of HP-uninfected pure SRCC.

References

1. Torre LA, Bray F, Siegel RL, et al. Global cancer statistics, 2012. CA Cancer J Clin. 2015;65:87–108.
2. Polk DB, Peek RM Jr. *Helicobacter pylori*: gastric cancer and beyond. Nat Rev Cancer. 2010;10:403–14.
3. Plummer M, Franceschi S, Vignat J, et al. Global burden of gastric cancer attributable to *Helicobacter pylori*. Int J Cancer. 2015;136:487–90.
4. Lee YC, Chiang TH, Chou CK, Tu YK, et al. Association between *Helicobacter pylori* eradication and gastric cancer incidence: a systematic review and meta-analysis. Gastroenterology. 2016;150:1113–24.
5. Rokkas T, Rokka A, Portincasa P. A systematic review and meta-analysis of the role of *Helicobacter pylori* eradication in preventing gastric cancer. Ann Gastroenterol. 2017;30:414–23.
6. The Editorial Board of the Cancer Statistics in Japan. Cancer statistics in Japan 2016. 2017.
7. Tsuda M, Asaka M, Kato M, et al. Effect of *Helicobacter pylori* eradication therapy against gastric cancer in Japan. Helicobacter. 2017;22:e12415.
8. Matsuo T, Ito M, Takata S, Tanaka S, et al. Low prevalence of *Helicobacter pylori*-negative gastric cancer among Japanese. Helicobacter. 2011;16:415–9.
9. Yamamoto Y, Fujisaki J, Omae M, et al. *Helicobacter pylori*-negative gastric cancer: characteristics and endoscopic findings. Dig Endosc. 2015;27:551–61.
10. Fitzgerald RC, Hardwick R, Huntsman D, et al. Hereditary diffuse gastric cancer: updated consensus guideline for clinical management and directions for future research. J Med Genet. 2010;47:436–44.
11. Cutsem EV, Sagaert X, Topal B, et al. Gastric Cancer. Lancet. 2016;388:2654–64.
12. Neumann WL, Coss E, Rugge M, Genta RM. Autoimmune atrophic gastritis: pathogenesis, pathology and management. Nat Rev Gastroenterol Hepatol. 2013;10:529–41.
13. Park JY, Lam-Himlin D, Vemulapalli R. Review of autoimmune metaplastic atrophic gastritis. Gastrointest Endosc. 2013;77:284–92.
14. Toh BH. Diagnosis and classification of autoimmune gastritis. Autoimmun Rev. 2014;13(4–5):459–62.
15. The Cancer Genome Atlas Research Network, Bass A, Thorsson V, Shmulevich B, et al. Comprehensive molecular characterization of gastric adenocarcinoma. Nature. 2014;513:202–9.
16. Van Beek J, Zur Hausen A, Kranenbarg EK, et al. EBV-positive gastric adenocarcinoma: a distinct clinicopathologic entity with a low frequency of lymph node involvement. J Clin Oncol. 2004;22:664–70.
17. Oliveira C, Pinheiro H, Figueiredo J, et al. Familial gastric cancer: genetic susceptibility, pathology, and implications for management. Lancet Oncol. 2015;16:e60–70.
18. Hansford S, Kaurah P, Li-Chang H, et al. Hereditary diffuse gastric cancer syndrome: CDH1 mutation and beyond. JAMA Oncol. 2015;1:23–32.
19. Horiuchi Y, Fujisaki J, Yamamoto N, et al. Biological behavior of the intramucosal *Helicobacter pylori*-negative undifferentiated-type early gastric cancer: comparison with *Helicobacter pylori*-positive early gastric cancer. Gastric Cancer. 2016;19:160–5.
20. Kiso M, Yoshihara M, Ito M, et al. Characteristics of gastric cancer in negative test of serum anti-*Helicobacter pylori* antibody and pepsinogen test: a multicenter study. Gastric Cancer. 2017;20:764–71.
21. Horiuchi Y, Fujisaki J, Ishizuka N, et al. Study of clinical factors involved in *Helicobacter pylori*-uninfected, undifferentiated-type early gastric cancer. Digestion. 2017;96:213–9.
22. Ono S, Kato M, Suzuki M, et al. Frequency of *Helicobacter pylori*-negative gastric cancer and gastric mucosal atrophy in a Japanese endoscopic submucosal dissection series including histological, endoscopic and serological atrophy. Digestion. 2012;86:59–65.

23. Van der Post RS, Vogelaar IP, Carneiro F, et al. Hereditary diffuse gastric cancer: updated clinical guideline with an emphasis on germline CDH1 mutation carriers. J Med Genet. 2015;52:316–74.
24. Carneiro F, Huntsman DG, Smyrk TC, et al. Model of the early development of diffuse gastric cancer in E-cadherin mutation carriers and its implication for patient screening. J Pathol. 2004;203:681–7.
25. Machado JC, Oliveira C, Carvalho R, et al. E-cadherin gene (CDH1) promoter methylation as the second hit in sporadic diffuse gastric cancer. Oncogene. 2001;20:1525–8.
26. Corso G, Carvalho J, Marrelli D, et al. Somatic mutations and deletions of the E-cadherin gene predict poor survival of patients with gastric cancer. J Clin Oncol. 2013;31:868–75.
27. Cho SY, Park JW, Liu Y, et al. Sporadic early-onset diffuse gastric cancers have a high frequency of somatic CDH1 alterations, but a low frequency of somatic RHOA mutations compared with late-onset cancers. Gastroenterology. 2017;153:536–49.
28. Humar B, Blair V, Charlton A, et al. E-cadherin deficiency initiates gastric signet-ring cell carcinoma in mice and man. Cancer Res. 2009;69:2050–6.
29. Mimata A, Fukamachi H, Eishi Y, et al. Loss of E-cadherin in mouse gastric epithelial cells induces signet ring-like cells, a possible precursor lesion of diffuse gastric cancer. Cancer Sci. 2011;102:942–50.
30. Hayakawa Y, Ariyama H, Stancikova J, et al. Mist1 expressing gastric stem cells maintain the normal and neoplastic gastric epithelium and are supported by a perivascular stem cell niche. Cancer Cell. 2015;28:800–14.
31. Ranzani GN, Luinetti O, Padovan LS, et al. p53 gene mutations and protein nuclear accumulation are early events in intestinal type gastric cancer but late events in diffuse type. Cancer Epidemiol Biomark Prev. 1995;4:223–31.
32. Shimada S, Mimata A, Sekine M, et al. Synergistic tumor suppressor activity of E-cadherin and p53 in a conditional mouse model of metastatic diffuse-type gastric cancer. Gut. 2012;61:344–53.

Chapter 5
Role of Alcohol and Metabolic Diseases in Colorectal Carcinogenesis

Tetsuji Takayama, Yasushi Sato, and Naoki Muguruma

Abstract Alcohol consumption was significantly associated with a risk of colorectal cancer with a relative risk ranging from 1.10 to 1.44 depending on the amount of intake. However, light intake of alcohol was not associated with incidence of colorectal cancer. Metabolic syndrome was also significantly associated with a risk of colorectal cancer with a relative risk ranging from 1.25 to 1.41. Of the four components of metabolic syndrome, dysglycemia and obesity were particularly associated with colorectal cancer risk. High levels of serum triglyceride were associated with increased colorectal cancer risk. However, there was no apparent association between raised blood pressure and colorectal cancer risk.

Keywords Alcohol · Metabolic syndrome · Colorectal cancer · Relative risk Dysglycemia · Obesity

It is widely recognized that the development of colorectal cancer is closely associated with lifestyle factors including diet, alcohol consumption, and metabolic syndrome. There is considerable evidence that red and processed meat, alcoholic beverages, excess body and abdominal fat, and low adult height are associated with an increased risk of colorectal cancer, and that this risk can be mitigated by physical activity and dietary fiber intake. In addition, metabolic disorders, including metabolic syndrome, which is characterized by obesity, hyperglycemia, dyslipidemia, and hypertension, are also associated with colorectal cancer.

In this review, we summarize the risk of alcohol consumption and metabolic syndrome for colorectal cancer and the postulated mechanisms of the relationship of alcohol consumption and metabolic disorders with colorectal carcinogenesis.

T. Takayama (✉) · N. Muguruma
Department of Gastroenterology and Oncology, Institutes of Biomedical Sciences, Tokushima University Graduate School, Tokushima, Japan
e-mail: takayama@tokushima-u.ac.jp

Y. Sato
Department of Community Medicine for Gastroenterology and Oncology, Institutes of Biomedical Sciences, Tokushima University Graduate School, Tokushima, Japan

H. Yoshiji, K. Kaji (eds.), *Alcoholic/Non-Alcoholic Digestive Diseases*,
https://doi.org/10.1007/978-981-13-1465-0_5

5.1 Colorectal Cancer Risk Attributable to Alcohol

It is well known that alcohol intake increases the risk of cancers of the oral cavity, pharynx, larynges, esophagus, and liver. Various cohort studies and randomized control trials have investigated the relationship between alcohol consumption and colorectal carcinogenesis. Meta-analyses by the World Cancer Research Fund (WCRF) in 2007 and International Agency for Research on Cancer (IARC) in 2010 reported that alcohol intake increases the risk of the five aforementioned cancers as well as the risk of colorectal and female breast cancer [1, 2].

In 2015, Vieira and colleagues conducted an update of the WCRFs 2007 meta-analysis [3]. The updated analysis, which included 14 studies comprising 12,051 subjects revealed that each additional 10 g/day of alcohol (ethanol) consumed increased the risk of colorectal cancer with a relative risk of 1.07 (95% CI 1.05–1.09) (Table 5.1). Ten grams of ethanol is equivalent to approximately 350 mL of beer, 125 mL of wine, 30 mL of liquor (distilled spirits), and 70 mL of Japanese sake. A sex-stratified analysis showed an increased risk in men and a marginally significant risk in women. The meta-analysis revealed that each 10 g/day alcohol intake increased the risks of colon cancer with a relative risk of 1.08 (95% CI 1.07–1.10) and the risk of rectal cancer with a relative risk of 1.08 (95% CI 1.07–1.10). Bagnardi and colleagues conducted a meta-analysis of 66 studies and 41,715 subjects to determine the risk of colorectal cancer associated with alcohol intake [4]. Moderate and heavy drinking, but not light drinking, was associated with colorectal cancer; i.e., the relative risks for moderate and heavy drinking were 1.17 (95% CI 1.11–1.24) and 1.44 (95% CI 1.25–1.65), respectively. Of note, when the risk was evaluated in men and women separately, the risk was significantly higher in men than women, and there was no significant effect of alcohol in women. In addition, Choi and colleagues reported a meta-analysis of 16 studies comprising 5,815,523 subjects to determine the cancer risk associated with light alcohol drinking [5]. Interestingly, very light drinking (≤0.5 drinks/day; 1 drink being equivalent to 12.5 g of ethanol or 355 mL of beer) or light drinking (≤1 drink/day) was not associated with the incidence of cancers of most organs. However, light drinking significantly increased the risk of colorectal cancer: relative risk was 1.04 (1.01–1.04) overall; 1.06 (1.01–1.11) for men and 1.02 (0.98–1.02) for women. Moderate

Table 5.1 Meta-analysis for the risk of colorectal cancers attributable to alcohol intake

Author	Alcohol consumption	Relative risk (95% CI)	No. of studies	No. of subjects	*p*-value	Year
Vieira, et al. [3]	Each additional 10 g/day	1.07 (1.05–1.09)	14	12,051	<0.01	2017
Bagnardi, et al. [4]	Moderate drinker	1.17 (1.1–1.24)	66	41,715	<0.01	2015
	Heavy drinker	1.44 (1.25–1.65)			<0.01	
Choi, et al. [5]	Very light drinker	1.10 (0.94–0.28)	16	5,815,523	N.S.	2018
	Light drinker	1.04 (1.01–1.04)			<0.05	
	Moderate drinker	1.10 (1.03–1.19)			<0.05	

N.S. Not significant

drinking (1–2 drinks/day) further increased the risk of colorectal cancer associated with alcohol intake: 1.10 (1.03–1.19) overall; 1.19 (1.06–1.35) for men and 1.04 (0.95–1.013) for women.

5.2 Risk for Precancerous Lesions in the Colorectum Attributable to Alcohol

It is widely accepted that a majority of colorectal cancers develop from colorectal adenoma, a precancerous lesion, with cumulative genetic abnormalities and morphological changes (adenoma-carcinoma sequence). Recently, the serrated pathway has been reported, as an alternative pathway, attracting a considerable attention. Serrated polyps comprise three types of polyps (sessile serrated adenoma/polyp, SSA/P; traditional serrated adenoma, TSA; and hyperplastic polyp, HP) that can develop into cancers [6]. Cancers from the serrated pathway account for approximately 15–30% of colorectal cancers. Of these, SSA/P is predominantly located in the right-side colon, and is considered to be a precursor of right-side colon cancer.

Several case–control studies have examined the association between alcohol consumption and the risk of adenomas. However, it remains unclear as to whether low-dose alcohol intake promotes or inhibits adenoma formation [3, 4]. A recent meta-analysis by Zhu et al. showed that alcohol intake was associated with a 17% increased risk for colorectal adenomas as compared with non-drinkers or occasional alcohol drinkers [7]. Moreover, they demonstrated a dose-dependent association between alcohol intake and the estimated relative risks for colorectal adenomas; i.e., the estimated relative risks associated with alcohol consumption at 10, 25, 50, and 100 g/day were 1.02 (95% CI 0.89–1.16), 1.06 (95% CI 0.92–1.20), 1.16 (95% CI 1.02–1.33), and 1.61 (95% CI 1.42–1.84), respectively. Ben and colleagues also performed a meta-analysis on the risk of colorectal adenomas and similarly reported that alcohol intake was closely associated with colorectal adenoma risk [8]. On the other hand, Bailie and colleagues reported a meta-analysis of 14 studies to determine the risk of serrated polyps in relation to *lifestyle*, which revealed a significant risk for serrated polyps in subjects with high alcohol consumption relative to low consumption [9]. Likewise, the relative risk of SSA/P in high alcohol consumption was 1.85 (95% CI 1.03–3.32).

5.3 Developmental Mechanism of Colorectal Cancer Attributable to Alcohol

Colorectal polyps (adenoma) are recognized as a precancerous lesion; thus, increased risk of colorectal cancer associated with alcohol intake may be associated with an increased risk of precancerous adenoma and serrated polyps, and several underlying mechanisms have been proposed. First, alcohol hinders the absorption of folic acid and calcium which both reportedly have anti-carcinogenic effects [10, 11]. Second, alcohol is metabolized into acetaldehydes in the colon, due to the high alcohol dehydrogenase activity of intestinal microflora, and high concentrations of acetaldehydes are known to promote the development of colorectal polyps. Alcohol and acetaldehydes have also been shown to exert carcinogenic effects on the colorectum in animals, which may be explained by the fact that alcohol and acetaldehyde induce DNA hypomethylation [12]. Acetaldehyde is also reported to alter DNA integrity and stability and thereby can affect the expression of oncogenes and tumor suppressor genes [13]. Moreover, alcohol and acetaldehyde are reported to suppress tumor immune surveillance.

5.4 Metabolic Syndrome and Colorectal Cancer Risk

Metabolic syndrome is a clustering of conditions comprising obesity, blood lipid abnormality, hyperglycemia, and high blood pressure. There are several diagnostic criteria for metabolic syndrome, including those of the World Health Organization (WHO) [14], National Cholesterol Education Program (NCEP) [15], International Diabetes Federation (IDF) [16], and Japan [17]. The criteria were similar although there were minor differences for each component parameter (Table 5.2).

Table 5.2 Criteria for metabolic syndrome

	WHO criteria [14]	NCEP criteria [15]	IDF criteria [16]	Japanese criteria [17]
Obesity	Waist/hip ratio (WHR) Men > 0.9 Women > 0.85 and/or BMI > 30 kg/m^2	Central obesity (BMI > 30 kg/m^2)	Waist circumference Men ≥ 94 cm Women ≥ 80 cm	Waist circumference Men ≥ 85 cm Women ≥ 90 cm
Dyslipidemia	high TG ≥ 150 mg/dL and/or low HDL-C Men < 35 mg/dL Women < 39 mg/dL	high TG ≥ 150 mg/dL and/or low HDL-C Men < 40 mg/dL Women < 50 mg/dL	high TG ≥ 150 mg/dL and/or low HDL-C Men < 40 mg/dL Women < 50 mg/dL	high TG ≥ 150 mg/dL and/or low HDL-C Men < 35 mg/dL Women < 40 mg/dL
Raised blood pressure	≥140/90 mmHg	≥130/85 mmHg	≥130/85 mmHg	≥130/85 mmHg
Glucose intolerance	FPG ≥ 110 mg/dL and/or PG after load ≥200 mg/dL	FPG ≥ 110 mg/dL	FPG ≥ 100 mg/dL	FPG ≥ 110 mg/dL
Others	Albuminuria ≥ 20mg/gCr			

WHO World Health Organization, *NCEP* National Cholesterol Education Program, *IDF* International Diabetes Federation, *BMI* body mass index, *TG* triglyceride, *HDL-C* high density lipoprotein-cholesterol, *FPG* fasting plasma glucose, *PG* plasma glucose

Table 5.3 Meta-analysis for the risk of colorectal cancers attributable to metabolic syndrome

Author	Category	Relative risk (95% CI)	No. of studies	No. of cases	*p*-value	Year
Esposito et al. [18]	Men	1.25 (1.19–1.32)	12	4814	<0.01	2012
	Women	1.34 (1.09–1.64)	10	3045	<0.01	
Jinjuvadia et al. [19]		1.34[a] (1.24–1.44)	18	703,992	<0.01	2013
Esposito et al. [20]	Men	1.33 (1.18–1.50)	15	6344	0.029	2013
	Women	1.41 (1.18–1.70)	14	4312	<0.01	

95% CI, 95% confidence interval
[a]Neoplasia including colorectal cancer and adenoma

5.5 Colorectal Cancer Risk Attributable to Metabolic Syndrome

Three meta-analyses to date have analyzed the impact of metabolic syndrome on colorectal cancer risk (Table 5.3). Esposito and colleagues performed a meta-analysis of 12 studies comprising 7859 cases (4814 men and 3045 women) [18]. In men, the presence of metabolic syndrome was associated with liver (relative risk 1.43, $p < 0.0001$), colorectal (1.25, $p < 0.01$), and bladder cancer (1.10, $p = 0.013$). In woman, the presence of metabolic syndrome was associated with endometrial (1.61, $p = 0.001$), pancreatic (1.58, $p < 0.0001$), breast postmenopausal (1.56, $p = 0.017$), and colorectal (1.34, $p = 0.006$) cancer. They also analyzed cancer mortality and found that the relative risk for death due to colorectal cancer in subjects with metabolic syndrome was 1.61 (1.28–2.01) ($p < 0.0001$). Jinjuvadia and colleagues performed a meta-analysis of 18 studies that included 703,992 cases [19]. The overall relative risk for colorectal neoplasms (adenoma or cancer) was 1.34 (95% CI 1.24–1.44). A subgroup analyses for men and women revealed relative risks of 1.31 (95% CI 1.19–1.44) and 1.32 (95% CI 1.11–1.56), respectively. A subgroup analysis of the 687,413 cases showed that the relative risk of colorectal cancer in those with metabolic syndrome was 1.30 (95% CI 1.18–1.43). Moreover, Esposito and colleagues reported a meta-analysis of 15 studies comprising 10,656 cases (6344 men and 4312 women) to analyze the association between metabolic syndrome and colorectal cancer [20]. The relative risk for colorectal cancer associated with metabolic syndrome was 1.33 (95% CI 1.18–1.50) for men and 1.41 (1.18–1.70) for women. Moreover, the relative risk for mortality due to colorectal cancer associated with metabolic syndrome was 1.36 (1.25–1.48) for men and 1.16 (1.03–1.30) for women. In these three meta-analyses, the relative risks of colorectal cancer incidence in subjects with metabolic syndrome were very similar (1.25–1.43).

5.6 Risk for Precancerous Lesions in the Colorectum Attributable to Metabolic Syndrome

A meta-analysis of 8 studies with 21,474 cases investigated the risk of colorectal adenoma in patients with metabolic syndrome. In this analysis, metabolic syndrome increased the risk of colorectal adenoma by 37% (relative risk 1.37, 95% CI

1.26–1.49) [18]. Moreover, Morita and colleagues performed a case–control study consisting of 756 patients with metabolic syndrome and 1756 control subjects to evaluate the risk of colorectal adenomas [21]. The metabolic syndrome was found to be associated with a moderately increased risk of colorectal adenomas. Increased risk was more evident for proximal than distal colon or rectal adenomas. Kim et al. also performed a large Korean cross-sectional study and found that metabolic syndrome increased the risk of colorectal adenoma, particularly proximal lesions, multiple adenomas, and advanced adenomas [22]. Thus, the metabolic syndrome increases the risk of colorectal adenoma as well as colorectal cancers.

5.7 Four Components of Metabolic Syndrome and Colorectal Cancer Risk

Regarding the four components of metabolic syndrome, there is a growing body of evidence indicating that dysglycemia and obesity are associated with the risk of colorectal cancer. However, it remains unclear as to whether dyslipidemia and elevated blood pressure are associated with colorectal cancer risk. Esposito and colleagues conducted a meta-analysis to compare the relative risk of colorectal cancer among subjects with full metabolic syndrome versus each of the individual four components [18]. The risk of colorectal cancer associated with full metabolic syndrome was similar to that with dysglycemia, and higher than that with obesity. Thus, it appears that dysglycemia is the most important factor for colorectal cancer risk among the four components of metabolic syndrome.

1. *Dysglycemia and colorectal cancer risk*

   Many studies have investigated the risk of colorectal cancer risks in subjects with dysglycemia, defined as diabetes mellitus (DM), impaired fasting plasma glucose (FPG), or impaired glucose tolerance. Guraya performed a meta-analysis of eight studies comprising 113,868 type 2 DM (T2DM) patients and 810,764 non-T2DM subjects to investigate the association between T2DM and colorectal cancer risk [23]. A significant positive correlation between T2DM and colorectal cancer was demonstrated, with a relative risk of 1.22 (95% CI 1.01–1.49). The relative risk of colorectal cancer in women (1.22; 95% CI 1.01–0.149) was higher than that in men (1.17; 95% CI 1.00–1.37). Luo and colleagues performed a meta-analysis of 29 studies with 209,924 DM patients and 2,414,214 non-DM subjects to determine the risk of colorectal neoplasia (cancer and adenoma) [24]. DM was shown to be a significant risk factor for colorectal neoplasia (relative risk 1.35, 95% CI 1.28–1.42). A subgroup analysis revealed that the risk increased significantly for both colorectal cancer (relative risk 1.37, 95% CI 1.30–1.45) and adenoma (relative risk 1.26, 95% CI 1.11–1.44). Moreover, Shi and colleagues performed a meta-analysis to investigate the dose-response relationship between FPG and colorectal cancer [25]. The relative risk for colorectal cancer per 20 mg/dl increase in FPG was 1.015 (95% CI 1.012–1.019, $p = 0.000$), indicating a clear linear dose-response relationship.

Regarding the prediabetic status, Huang and associates performed a meta-analysis of 16 studies comprising 891,426 cases to evaluate the colorectal cancer risk in prediabetic subjects [26]. Prediabetes was associated with an increased risk of cancer overall (RR 1.15; 95% CI 1.06, 1.23). A subgroup analysis showed a significant relative risk of stomach/colorectal cancer (relative risk 1.55, 1.15–2.09).

2. *Obesity and colorectal cancer risk*

   A number of studies have investigated the association between obesity and colorectal cancer. Dong and colleagues performed a meta-analysis of 19 studies comprising 1,343,560 cases and showed that greater waist circumference was significantly associated with an increased risk of colorectal cancer (relative risk 1.42, 95% CI 1.30–1.55) [27]. Similarly, a meta-analysis by Ma and colleagues consisting of 41 studies and 8,115,689 participants showed that the relative risk of colorectal cancer among obese versus subjects with normal BMI was 1.334 (95% CI 1.253–1.420) [28]. They also reported a meta-analysis of 13 studies with 817,449 participants showing that the relative risk of colorectal cancer for subjects with high versus low waist circumference was 1.455 (95% CI 1.327–1.596). In addition, Wang and colleagues investigated the association between BMI and cancer incidence in a meta-analysis of 23 studies in men and 20 studies in women, and showed that the relative risks for colorectal cancer (per 5 kg/m^2 increase in BMI) was 1.13 (1.10–1.17) and 1.06 (1.03–1.09), respectively [29]. The relative risk in obese men was significantly higher than that in obese women ($p = 0.011$).

3. *Dyslipidemia and/or raised blood pressures and colorectal cancer risk*

   It is unclear whether dyslipidemia is associated with colorectal cancer. However, meta-analyses have shown that high levels of serum triglyceride are associated with increased colorectal cancer risk [30–32]. Other lipids including cholesterol, VLDL, HDL, LDL may not affect the risk of colorectal cancer. There is no apparent association between raised blood pressure and colorectal cancer risk.

5.8 Developmental Mechanism of Colorectal Cancer Attributable to Metabolic Syndrome

The detailed mechanism underlying the elevated risk of colorectal cancer in patients with metabolic syndrome has not been clarified. One of the factors involved, metabolic syndrome, may serve as a surrogate marker for other factors associated with colorectal cancer risk such as high dietary fat intake, high calorie diets, and physical inactivity. Regarding the molecular mechanism of colorectal carcinogenesis in metabolic syndrome, the following has been proposed.

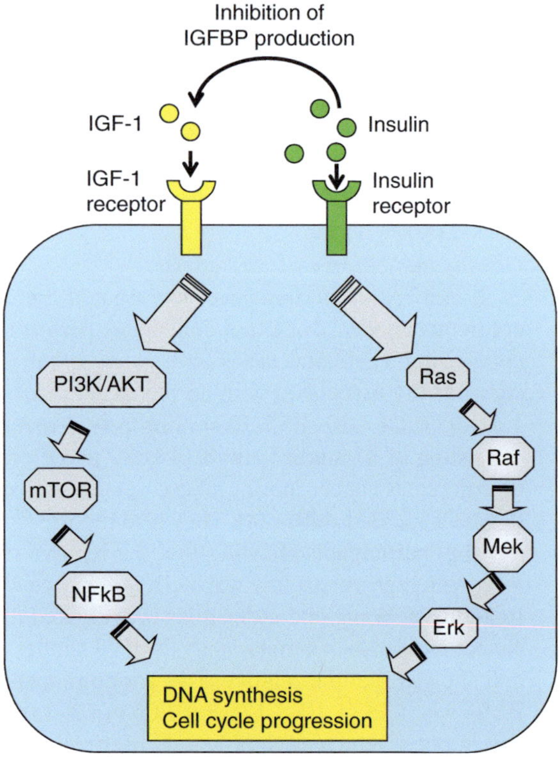

Fig. 5.1 Hyperinsulinemia and development of colorectal cancer. High levels of insulin induce DNA synthesis and cell cycle progression via the Ras/Raf/Mek/Erk and PIK3/Akt/mTOR pathways. Hyperinsulinemia inhibits insulin growth factor binding protein (IGFBP) production, and resulting elevation of free IGF-1 also promotes DNA synthesis and cell cycle progression in the same signal transduction

1. Dysregulation of growth factors such as Insulin growth factor-1 (IGF-1) and insulin (Fig. 5.1)

   Under conditions of insulin resistance, which is a core component of metabolic syndrome, beta cells of Langerhans islands in the pancreas produce an excess of insulin, thereby leading to hyperinsulinemia. High levels of insulin induce cell proliferation, angiogenesis, invasion, and anti-apoptosis in colorectal epithelia as well as other cells through the Ras/Raf/Mek/Erk and PIK3/Akt/mTOR pathways [33, 34]. Moreover, insulin inhibits the production of IGF-1 binding protein, and free IGF-1, resulting from inhibition of IGF-1–binding proteins, binds to IGF-1 receptors leading to cell proliferation, angiogenesis, invasion, and anti-apoptosis via similar signal transduction pathways.
2. Inflammatory cytokines

   Inflammatory cytokines produced by adipocytes and infiltrating macrophages stimulate signal transduction leading to DNA synthesis and cell cycle progression [35]. Interleukin-6 (IL-6) binds to IL-6 receptors and stimulates cell proliferation through the JAK/STAT pathway and/or through Ras/Raf/Mek/Erk and PIK3/Akt/mTOR pathways [36]. Tumor necrosis factor-alpha (TNF-alpha) may stimulate cell proliferation and survival via AP-1 and the NF-kappaB signaling pathway [37].
3. It has been reported that hyperglycemia induces the formation of reactive oxygen species (ROS), and high levels of ROS are likely to induce DNA damage [38].

5.9 Epilogue

Alcohol is widely consumed worldwide. Although consumption of a modest amount of alcohol is not associated with harmful effects, and may in fact be beneficial, excessive alcohol consumption poses health hazards including an increased risk of colorectal cancers. The incidence of metabolic syndrome is increasing both in developed countries and developing countries, which is also associated with an increased risk of various many diseases including colorectal cancer. The findings reported herein underscore the importance of lifestyle factors, such as eating an appropriate diet and limiting alcohol consumption, for overall optimal health.

References

1. World Cancer Research Fund/American Institute for Cancer Research. Food, nutrition, physical activity, and the prevention of cancer: a global perspective. Washington: American Institute for Cancer Research; 2007.
2. IARC Working Group. IARC monographs on the evaluation of carcinogenic risk to humans: alcohol consumption and ethylcalbamate, vol. 96. Lyon: International Agency of Research on Cancer; 2010.
3. Vieira AR, Abar L, Chan DSM, Vingeliene S, et al. Foods and beverages and colorectal cancer risk: a systematic review and meta-analysis of cohort studies, an update of the evidence of the WCRF-AICR continuous update project. Ann Oncol. 2017;28(8):1788–802.
4. Bagnardi V, Rota M, Botteri E, et al. Alcohol consumption and site-specific cancer risk: a comprehensive dose–response meta-analysis. Br J Cancer. 2015;112:580–93.
5. Choi YJ, Myung SK, Lee JH. Light alcohol drinking and risk of cancer: a meta-analysis of cohort studies. Cancer Res Treat. 2018;50(2):474–87.
6. Snover DC, Ahnen DJ, Burt RW. Serrated polyps of the colon and rectum and serrated polyposis. In: Bosman FT, Carneiro F, Hruban RH, Theise ND, editors. WHO classification of tumours of the digestive system. Lyon: IARC; 2010. p. 160–5.
7. Zhu JZ, Wang YM, Zhou QY, et al. Systematic review with meta-analysis: alcohol consumption and the risk of colorectal adenoma. Aliment Pharmacol Ther. 2014;40(4):325–37.
8. Ben Q, Wang L, Liu J, et al. Alcohol drinking and the risk of colorectal adenoma: a dose-response meta-analysis. Eur J Cancer Prev. 2015;24(4):286–95.
9. Bailie L, Loughrey MB, Coleman HG. Lifestyle risk factors for serrated colorectal polyps: a systematic review and meta-analysis. Gastroenterology. 2017;152(1):92–104.
10. Kennedy DA, Stern SJ, Moretti M, et al. Folate intake and the risk of colorectal cancer: a systematic review and meta-analysis. Cancer Epidemiol. 2011;35(1):2–10.
11. Huncharek M, Muscat J, Kupelnick B. Colorectal cancer risk and dietary intake of calcium, vitamin D, and dairy products: a meta-analysis of 26,335 cases from 60 observational studies. Nutr Cancer. 2009;61(1):47–69.
12. Pöschl G, Stickel F, Wang XD, et al. Alcohol and cancer: genetic and nutritional aspects. Proc Nutr Soc. 2004;63(1):65–71.
13. Lamarche F, Gonthier B, Signorini N, et al. Impact of ethanol and acetaldehyde on DNA and cell viability of cultured neurones. Cell Biol Toxicol. 2004;20(6):361–74.
14. Alberti KG, Zimmet PZ. Definition, diagnosis and classification of diabetes mellitus and its complications. Part 1: diagnosis and classification of diabetes mellitus provisional report of a WHO consultation. Diabet Med. 1998;15:539–53.
15. Expert Panel on Detection, Evaluation, and Treatment of High Blood Cholesterol in Adults. Executive summary of the third report of the national cholesterol education program (NCEP)

expert panel on detection, evaluation, and treatment of high blood cholesterol in adults (adult treatment panel III). JAMA. 2001;285(19):2486–97.
16. Alberti KG, Zimmet P, Shaw J, IDF Epidemiology Task Force Consensus Group. The metabolic syndrome–a new worldwide definition. Lancet. 2005;366(9491):1059–62.
17. Matsuzawa Y. Committee to evaluate diagnostic standards for metabolic syndrome: definition and the diagnostic standard for metabolic syndrome. Nippon Naika Gakkai Zasshi. 2005;94:794–809. (in Japanese).
18. Esposito K, Chiodini P, Colao A, et al. Metabolic syndrome and risk of cancer: a systematic review and meta-analysis. Diabetes Care. 2012;35(11):2402–11.
19. Jinjuvadia R, Lohia P, Jinjuvadia C, et al. The association between metabolic syndrome and colorectal neoplasm: systemic review and meta-analysis. J Clin Gastroenterol. 2013;47(1):33–44.
20. Esposito K, Chiodini P, Capuano A, et al. Colorectal cancer association with metabolic syndrome and its components: a systematic review with meta-analysis. Endocrine. 2013;44(3):634–47.
21. Morita T, Tabata S, Mineshita M, et al. The metabolic syndrome is associated with increased risk of colorectal adenoma development: the self-defense forces health study. Asian Pac J Cancer Prev. 2005;6(4):485–9.
22. Kim JH, Lim YJ, Kim YH, et al. Is metabolic syndrome a risk factor for colorectal adenoma? Cancer Epidemiol Biomark Prev. 2007;16:1543–6.
23. Guraya SY. Association of type 2 diabetes mellitus and the risk of colorectal cancer: a meta-analysis and systematic review. World J Gastroenterol. 2015;21(19):6026–31.
24. Luo S, Li JY, Zhao LN, Yu T, et al. Diabetes mellitus increases the risk of colorectal neoplasia: an updated meta-analysis. Clin Res Hepatol Gastroenterol. 2016;40(1):110–23.
25. Shi J, Xiong L, Li J, Cao H, et al. A linear dose-response relationship between fasting plasma glucose and colorectal cancer risk: systematic review and meta-analysis. Sci Rep. 2015;5:17591.
26. Huang Y, Cai X, Qiu M, et al. Prediabetes and the risk of cancer: a meta-analysis. Diabetologia. 2014;57(11):2261–9.
27. Dong Y, Zhou J, Zhu Y, et al. Abdominal obesity and colorectal cancer risk: systematic review and meta-analysis of prospective studies. Biosci Rep. 2017;37(6):BSR201745. (in press).
28. Ma Y, Yang Y, Wang F, et al. Obesity and risk of colorectal cancer: a systematic review of prospective studies. PLoS One. 2013;8(1):e53916.
29. Wang J, Yang DL, Chen ZZ, et al. Associations of body mass index with cancer incidence among populations, genders, and menopausal status: a systematic review and meta-analysis. Cancer Epidemiol. 2016;42:1–8.
30. Passarelli MN, Newcomb PA. Blood lipid concentrations and colorectal adenomas: a systematic review and meta-analysis of colonoscopy studies in Asia, 2000-2014. Am J Epidemiol. 2016;183(8):691–700.
31. Tian Y, Wang K, Li J, et al. The association between serum lipids and colorectal neoplasm: a systemic review and meta-analysis. Public Health Nutr. 2015;18(18):3355–70.
32. Yao X, Tian Z. Dyslipidemia and colorectal cancer risk: a meta-analysis of prospective studies. Cancer Causes Control. 2015;26(2):257–68.
33. Pollak M. The insulin and insulin-like growth factor receptor family in neoplasia: an update. Nat Rev Cancer. 2012;12(3):159–69.
34. Renehan AG, Frystyk J, Flyvbjerg A. Obesity and cancer risk: the role of the insulin-IGF axis. Trends Endocrinol Metab. 2006;17:328–36.
35. Kim S, Keku TO, Martin C, et al. Circulating levels of inflammatory cytokines and risk of colorectal adenomas. Cancer Res. 2008;68(1):323–8.
36. Neurath MF, Finotto S. IL-6 signaling in autoimmunity, chronic inflammation and inflammation-associated cancer. Cytokine Growth Factor Rev. 2011;22(2):83–9.
37. Balkwill F. Tumour necrosis factor and cancer. Nat Rev Cancer. 2009;9(5):361–71.
38. Othman EM, Leyh A, Stopper H. Insulin mediated DNA damage in mammalian colon cells and human lymphocytes in vitro. Mutat Res. 2013;745–746:34–9.

Part II
Alcoholic/Non-Alcoholic Liver Diseases

Chapter 6
Extracellular Vesicles in Alcoholic Liver Injury

Akiko Eguchi and Yoshiyuki Takei

Abstract Alcoholic liver disease (ALD) is one of the most common forms of chronic liver disease in the world; it is a major cause of chronic illness and mortality associated with alcohol over-consumption. ALD represents a broad spectrum of liver injury, such as hepatocyte cell death, liver inflammation, angiogenesis, and fibrosis leading to cirrhosis and hepatocellular carcinoma. Chronic ethanol consumption results in hepatic lipid accumulation and increases cell stress, which leads to inflammation and liver injury during the progression of ALD. It has been shown that crosstalk between hepatocytes and non-parenchymal cells is significantly important. The identifying factors that communicate stress signals from hepatocytes, and may initiate and perpetuate the inflammatory reaction responsible for liver injury and disease progression from steatohepatitis to cirrhosis may have a tremendous biomedical impact. Furthermore, the elucidation of these molecular mechanisms of crosstalk may allow for the identification of an individualized therapeutic approach in the treatment of patients with different stages of ALD and for the development of biomarkers to diagnose ALD progression. Recently, extracellular vesicles (EVs) have been identified as cell-to-cell communicators, the cellular contents of which contain proteins, lipids, and RNAs from stressed/activated cells and transfer this cellular payload to target cells. In this chapter, we will focus on current reports of EV function, how they are involved in the molecular pathogenesis of ALD, and EV biomarkers using EV composition.

Keywords Extracellular vesicles · Alcoholic liver injury · ALD · ASH · AH

A. Eguchi · Y. Takei (✉)
Department of Gastroenterology and Hepatology, Graduate School of Medicine, Mie University, Tsu, Japan
e-mail: akieguchi@clin.medic.mie-u.ac.jp; ytakei@clin.medic.mie-u.ac.jp

H. Yoshiji, K. Kaji (eds.), *Alcoholic/Non-Alcoholic Digestive Diseases*,
https://doi.org/10.1007/978-981-13-1465-0_6

6.1 Introduction

6.1.1 *Alcoholic Liver Injury*

Alcoholic liver disease (ALD) is the common cause of chronic liver disease in the world [1]. ALD represents a wide spectrum of liver injury ranging from alcoholic steatosis, alcoholic steatohepatitis (ASH), cirrhosis to liver failure and hepatocellular carcinoma [2]. In the process of ALD progression, hepatocyte damage, inflammation, fibrosis, and angiogenesis are key events and are closely interconnected [3], suggesting that multiple-hits involve in the progression of ALD. Current growing evidences show that extracellular vesicles (EVs) releasing from damaged hepatocytes or non-parenchymal cells contribute to the progression of liver diseases through activation of target cells, such as hepatic stellate cells and hepatic macrophages [4, 5]. Furthermore, EV composition, such as proteins and microRNAs (miRNAs), can be used to identify the degree of liver diseases including ALD/ASH [4, 6].

6.1.2 *Extracellular Vesicles (EVs)*

EVs are released from various cell types with their cell contents, such as proteins, non-coding RNAs, and lipids, in a highly regulated manner and circulated into the blood with high stability. Circulating EV levels are increased in many diseases due to up-regulation of EV release from damaged and activated cells, thus EVs including EV compositions will be able to use for biomarkers [7]. EVs are mainly categorized as exosomes or microparticles (MPs)/microvesicles. Exosomes are enclosed in the multi-vesicle body (MVB) and released from the cells in the endosomal pathway, whereas MPs are budded from the plasma membrane. Traditionally, their size was defined below 100–150 nm for exosomes and around 200–500 nm for MPs, but small vesicles (~100 nm) were identified as budding form as same as MPs [8]. As larger than nano-size, apoptotic bodies (above 1 μm) and oncosomes (1–10 μm) from cancer cells, which are budded from the plasma membrane, are also categorized in EVs [9]. In the molecular content, some of their composition may be different, CD63 for exosomes and annexin V for MPs, but traditionally identified molecules, such as CD81, CD9, or TSG101, are contained both in exosomes and MPs [8]. Lacking a clear categorization of EV type by size and contents, a new system of nomenclature has been proposed for studies lacking a detailed analysis of EV biogenesis whereby vesicles are grouped into one of two categories, small EVs or large EVs [9]. Notably, EVs are efficiently internalized into target cells and the subsequent transferring of their molecular composition, such as proteins, non-coding RNAs including microRNAs (miRNAs), messenger RNAs (mRNAs), DNA, and lipids, is a key mechanism by which EVs modulate cell signaling in target cells [8, 9], so called cell-to-cell communication. For instance, ligands on EVs bind to their specific receptor on the target cells and release encapsulated miRNAs, which in turn bind to target cell mRNA, thus altering the cell signaling pathway via translational suppression [10].

6.2 The Mechanism of EV Release and the Role of EVs in ALD/ASH

Circulating EV levels were increased in both animal models of ALD and human ALD patients. The source of the EVs was identified using EV composition, such as asialoglycoprotein receptor 1 (ASGPR1), vanin-1, and miR-122, which would indicate that a portion of the circulating EVs were derived from hepatocytes [4]. Supporting evidence that the liver releases hepatocyte-derived EVs (Hep-EVs) was directly confirmed when large quantities of EVs were found to be released from damaged hepatocytes isolated from alcoholic steatohepatitis (ASH) mice compared to control-diet mice [11]. Non-parenchymal cells also release EVs in ALD that are circulated in the blood. Liver EVs derived from hepatocytes and non-parenchymal cells contribute to the progression of ALD.

6.2.1 Hepatocyte-Derived Extracellular Vesicles (Hep-EVs)

Various pathways, including the activation of caspase and pho-kinase, as well as ER stress are involved in Hep-EV release [4, 11], resulting in Hep-EVs containing damage-associated cellular molecules, such as proteins, ligands, miRNAs, and mtDNAs, used in the activation of target cells (Fig. 6.1).

A significant amount of Hep-EVs, which contained CD40 ligand (CD40L), were released in a caspase-3-dependent-manner from HepG2 cells treated with EtOH and overexpressing cytochrome P450 2E1, which is related to ethanol metabolism [12]. CD40L containing Hep-EVs activated macrophages to the M1 type inflammatory phenotype through the activation of ERK, whereas Hep-EV macrophage activation was attenuated using a CD40L-specific antibody. In a chronic Lieber-DeCarli diet plus single binge ethanol feeding model, wild-type mice receiving a pan-caspase/Rho kinase inhibitor or with a genetic deletion of either CD40 ($CD40^{-/-}$) or the caspase-activating tumor necrosis factor-related apoptosis-inducing ligand (TRAIL) receptor ($TR^{-/-}$) were protected from ethanol induced liver injury due to the attenuation of macrophage infiltration. Macrophage activation with Hep-EVs was also observed in a different experimental model that isolated hepatocytes from an intragastric infusion model of ASH, which significantly released Hep-EVs in a caspase 3-dependent-manner and these Hep-EVs were internalized and activated primary hepatic macrophages into the inflammatory M1 type [11, 13]. In the chronic Lieber-DeCarli diet-plus single binge ethanol feeding model, mtDNA-enriched circulating

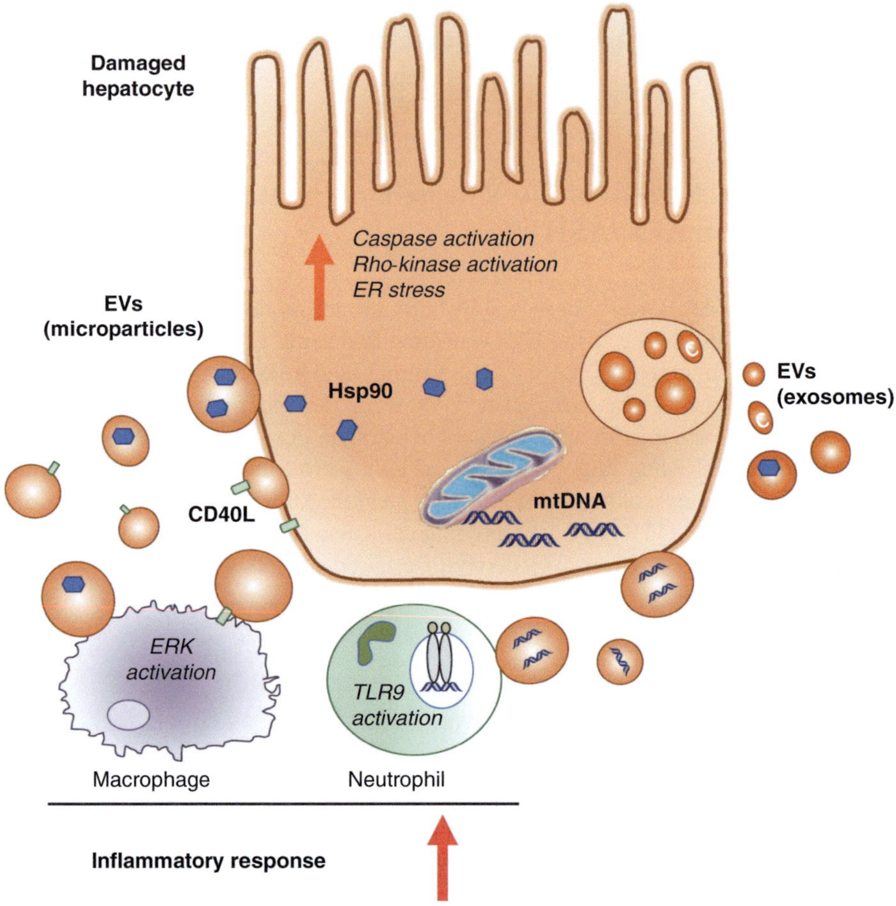

Fig. 6.1 Hepatocyte-derived EVs are cell-to-cell communicators for the progression of ALD. Hepatocyte-derived EVs (Hep-EVs), exosomes and microparticles, released from damaged hepatocytes activate target cells (hepatic macrophages, monocytes, neutrophils) via cell-to-cell communication. Hep-EVs contain unique molecular cargo, such as proteins and miRNAs, that reflects cellular damage/stress and this cargo modulates the activation of target cells

EVs were increased associated with the activation of hepatic ER stress and inflammatory responses, particularly the inflammasome [14]. Hepatocytes were the main source of mtDNA-enriched EVs, since mtDNA-enriched EVs were decreased in a hepatocyte-specific deletion of the protein kinase RNA-like ER kinase (*Perk*) gene in mice. mtDNA-enriched circulating EV levels, and the degree of neutrophil infiltration in the liver, were attenuated in transcriptional factor C/EBP homologous protein (*Chop*) KO mice, Jun-amino-terminal kinase 2 (*JNK2*) KO mice, or caspase-1 inhibitor treated mice, which is an ER stress-related gene, an ER stress-associated protein, or an inflammasome-associated gene, respectively. In an in vivo transfer EV assay, chronic ethanol fed mice injected with mtDNA-enriched circulating EVs induced neutrophilic inflammation through TLR9 activation. In chronic ethanol fed (Lieber-DeCarli diet) mice, which delivers a more mild liver pathology compared to the Lieber-DeCarli plus binge feeding model, circulating EVs (Hep-EVs plus other EVs) from ALD (ALD-EVs) were internalized via an in vivo transfer EV assay into the hepatocytes and Kupffer cells (KCs) of naïve mice which induced an increase of MCP-1 mRNA levels in hepatocytes and elevated inflammatory M1 type KCs and infiltrating monocytes [15]. Heat shock protein 90 (Hsp90) was highly enriched in ALD-EVs, as assessed by mass spectrometry analysis, and contributed to RAW macrophage activation associated with TNFα elevation. Conversely, macrophage activation was suppressed in RAW cells treated with a competitive inhibitor of Hsp90 plus ALD-EVs. These results suggest that Hep-EVs are an Hsp90 carrier and are involved in macrophage activation, since Hsp90 is a key player in macrophage activation as the literature has shown [16].

6.2.2 *Non-parenchymal Cell-Derived Extracellular Vesicles*

Hep-EVs from damaged hepatocytes were the major source of EVs in ASH mice (intra-gastric EtOH infusion), but non-parenchymal cells, such as hepatic macrophages, also released EVs associated with liver injury [11]. Indeed, alcohol-exposed monocytes, human primary monocytes, and THP-1 monocytic cells released miR-27a-enriched EVs [17]. miR-27a-enriched EVs stimulated naive monocytes into M2 macrophages associated with the up-regulation of IL-10 and TGF-β followed by increased monocyte phagocytosis. Circulating miR-27a-enriched EVs from AH patients polarize monocytes into an M2 phenotype associated with an elevation of IL-10.

6.3 EVs as Novel Biomarkers to Monitor Liver Injury in ALD/ASH

Various imaging modalities, such as ultrasound- and MR-based elastography, are increasingly being used for the assessment of liver fibrosis. However, liver biopsy still remains the gold standard in which to determine ALD staging with hepatocellular injury and hepatic inflammation. EVs have a key pathophysiological role in liver injury, as described in the previous sections, and EVs are remarkably stable in the blood during circulation, thus EVs, as well as EV composition, carry the potential to be developed into noninvasive biomarkers.

Growing evidence using animal models and human patients shows that the number of circulating EVs and liver-specific EV composition levels, such as asialoglycoprotein receptor 1 (ASGPR1), miR-122, and miR-192, are increased in various liver diseases including ALD, non-alcoholic steatohepatitis, viral hepatitis, and

Table 6.1 Summary of EV biomarkers in ALD

Increased EV composition	Source from cells	Source from mice (Model)	Source from human (Patients)	Ref.
CD40L	Hep-EVs (CYP2E1 overexpressing HepG2 cells)	Circulating EVs (chronic-plus single binge ethanol feeding)	Circulating EVs (AH patients)	[12]
Hsp90		Circulating EVs (chronic ethanol feeding)		[15]
mtDNA		Circulating EVs (chronic-plus single binge ethanol feeding)	Circulating EVs (chronic EAU with RD patients)	[14]
miR-27a	Monocyte-EVs (primary monocytes and THP-1 cells)		Circulating EVs (AH patients)	[17]
miR-30a		Circulating EVs (chronic ethanol feeding)	Circulating EVs (AH patients)	[19]
miR-29a, miR-340, let7f	Hep-EVs (isolated hepatocytes from ASH mice)	Circulating EVs (chronic intra-gastric infusion)	Circulating EVs (ALD patients)	[11]

EV extracellular vesicles, *ALD* alcoholic liver disease, *CD40L* CD40 ligand, *Hep-EV* hepatocyte-derived EV, *CYP2E1* cytochrome P450 2E1, *AH* alcoholic hepatitis, *mtDNA* mitochondrial DNA, *EAU* excessive alcohol use, *RD* recent excessive drinking, *Monocyte-EV* monocyte-derived EV, *ASH* alcoholic steatohepatitis

cirrhosis [4, 6, 18–20]. Circulating EV levels and liver specific EV composition levels may not be able to distinguish liver diseases by type, thus we need to identify specific EV composition to confirm ALD diagnosis. We introduce biomarkers, proteins, mtDNAs, and miRNAs in ALD/ASH, but focus exclusively on liver-specific proteins and miRNAs in this section (Table 6.1).

6.3.1 Ligands and Proteins

CD40L levels on circulating EVs were increased in alcoholic hepatitis patients compared to healthy individual or individuals who consume alcohol [12]. CD40L enriched-EVs were involved in macrophage activation. Using proteomic analysis, many proteins relating to the inflammatory response, cellular development, and cellular movement were enriched in circulating ALD-EVs from chronic ethanol feeding mice compared to circulating control-EVs [15]. One of the identified proteins was Hsp90, which induced macrophage activation, and high Hsp90 expression was validated in circulating ALD-EVs compared to control-EVs. Interestingly, at least ten proteins were only expressed in ALD-EVs and they were related to alcohol metabolism and redox regulation. These proteins are not yet validated in EVs from human alcoholic patients.

6.3.2 mtDNAs and miRNAs

mtDNAs levels in circulating EVs were higher in chronic-plus single binge ethanol feeding mice compared to pair-feeding mice, chronic ethanol feeding mice, or single binge ethanol feeding mice [14]. Furthermore, mtDNAs levels in circulating EVs were also elevated in chronic excessive alcohol use (EAU) with recent excessive drinking (RD) patients compared to EAU without RD patient or healthy controls. mtDNA-enriched EVs led to neutrophilia and liver injury. For miRNAs, miR-27a levels in circulating EVs were increased in AH patients compared to healthy controls [17]. miR-27a-enriched EVs mediated a polarization from monocytes to M2 type macrophage. Using firefly miRNA multiplex assay, seven miRNAs including miR-30a were significantly up-regulated and two miRNAs were significantly down-regulated in circulating ALD-EVs from chronic ethanol feeding mice compared to control-EVs from pair-feeding mice [19]. miR-30a had an excellent diagnostic value in ALD mice and miR-30a was significantly increased in alcoholic hepatitis patients compared to healthy controls. Using RNA-sequencing approach to assess miRNA composition in Hep-EVs released by hepatocytes isolated from the intra-gastric infusion model of ASH, nine miRNAs were significantly up-regulated and four miRNAs were significantly down-regulated in ASH Hep-EVs compared to control Hep-EVs [11]. miR-29a, miR-340, and let7f were increased in circulating EVs from ASH mice, but not in circulating EVs from bile duct ligation, NASH, and obese, indicating these miRNAs identify ASH. Three miRNAs were also elevated in ALD patients compared to non-alcoholics.

6.4 Conclusions

We have summarized some of the most recent and original studies investigating the biological function of EVs and their potential as biomarkers specific for ALD/ASH. In particular, many studies have pointed to the biological role of Hep-EVs released by stressed/damaged hepatocytes as key modulators for target cells as cell-to-cell communicator during ALD progression. According to many studies that looked into the biological role of EVs in different liver diseases—fatty liver, NASH, cirrhosis—some of the roles or release mechanisms of EVs are similar in ALD. For instance, mtDNA-enriched Hep-EVs were increased in NASH patients and mediated macrophage activation through TLR9 activation [21]. Damaged hepatocytes released Hep-EVs by lipotoxicity in a caspase3-dependent-manner and activated target cells [22], although EV composition was different in the process of target cell modulation. Since EVs have various biological roles in the progression of other liver diseases [5], we expect to identify other roles for EVs in ALD for future study. In addition, our work with EVs will contribute in the development of specific biomarkers for alcoholic liver injury.

Acknowledgments This work was partially supported by JSPS KAKENHI Grant Number JP16H06872 to AE and JSPS KAKENHI Grant Number JP17K09419 to YT.

Conflicts of Interest No potential conflict of interest relevant to this article was reported.

References

1. Rehm J, Samokhvalov AV, Shield KD. Global burden of alcoholic liver diseases. J Hepatol. 2013;59:160–8. https://doi.org/10.1016/j.jhep.2013.03.007.
2. Stickel F, Datz C, Hampe J, Bataller R. Pathophysiology and management of alcoholic liver disease: update 2016. Gut Liver. 2017;11:173–88. https://doi.org/10.5009/gnl16477.
3. Bocca C, Novo E, Miglietta A, Parola M. Angiogenesis and fibrogenesis in chronic liver diseases. Cell Mol Gastroenterol Hepatol. 2015;1:477–88. https://doi.org/10.1016/j.jcmgh.2015.06.011.
4. Hirsova P, Ibrahim SH, Verma VK, Morton LA, Shah VH, LaRusso NF, Gores GJ, Malhi H. Extracellular vesicles in liver pathobiology: small particles with big impact. Hepatology. 2016;64:2219–33. https://doi.org/10.1002/hep.28814.
5. Povero D, Feldstein AE. Novel molecular mechanisms in the development of non-alcoholic steatohepatitis. Diabetes Metab J. 2016;40:1–11. https://doi.org/10.4093/dmj.2016.40.1.1.
6. Szabo G, Momen-Heravi F. Extracellular vesicles in liver disease and potential as biomarkers and therapeutic targets. Nat Rev Gastroenterol Hepatol. 2017;14:455–66. https://doi.org/10.1038/nrgastro.2017.71.
7. Raposo G, Stoorvogel W. Extracellular vesicles: exosomes, microvesicles, and friends. J Cell Biol. 2013;200:373–83. https://doi.org/10.1083/jcb.201211138.
8. Yanez-Mo M, Siljander PR, Andreu Z, Zavec AB, Borras FE, Buzas EI, Buzas K, Casal E, Cappello F, Carvalho J, et al. Biological properties of extracellular vesicles and their physiological functions. J Extracell Vesicles. 2015;4:27066. https://doi.org/10.3402/jev.v4.27066.
9. Maas SLN, Breakefield XO, Weaver AM. Extracellular vesicles: unique intercellular delivery vehicles. Trends Cell Biol. 2017;27:172–88. https://doi.org/10.1016/j.tcb.2016.11.003.
10. Chen K, Rajewsky N. The evolution of gene regulation by transcription factors and microRNAs. Nat Rev Genet. 2007;8:93–103. https://doi.org/10.1038/nrg1990.
11. Eguchi A, Lazaro RG, Wang J, Kim J, Povero D, Willliams B, Ho SB, Starkel P, Schnabl B, Ohno-Machado L, et al. Extracellular vesicles released by hepatocytes from gastric infusion model of alcoholic liver disease contain a MicroRNA barcode that can be detected in blood. Hepatology. 2017;65:475–90. https://doi.org/10.1002/hep.28838.
12. Verma VK, Li H, Wang R, Hirsova P, Mushref M, Liu Y, Cao S, Contreras PC, Malhi H, Kamath PS, et al. Alcohol stimulates macrophage activation through caspase-dependent hepatocyte derived release of CD40L containing extracellular vesicles. J Hepatol. 2016;64:651–60. https://doi.org/10.1016/j.jhep.2015.11.020.
13. Eguchi A, Kim J, Ohno-Machado L, Tsukamoto H, Feldstein AE. Hepatocytes from mice on intragastric feeding model of alcoholic steatohepatitis release extracellular vesicles with specific microRNA cargo that modulate hepatic stellate cell and macrophage phenotype. Hepatology. 2015;62:266A–7A.
14. Cai Y, Xu MJ, Koritzinsky EH, Zhou Z, Wang W, Cao H, Yuen PS, Ross RA, Star RA, Liangpunsakul S, et al. Mitochondrial DNA-enriched microparticles promote acute-on-chronic alcoholic neutrophilia and hepatotoxicity. JCI Insight. 2017;2:92634. https://doi.org/10.1172/jci.insight.92634.
15. Saha B, Momen-Heravi F, Furi I, Kodys K, Catalano D, Gangopadhyay A, Haraszti R, Satishchandran A, Iracheta-Vellve A, Adejumo A, et al. Extracellular vesicles from mice with alcoholic liver disease carry a distinct protein cargo and induce macrophage activation via Hsp90. Hepatology. 2017;67(5):1986–2000. https://doi.org/10.1002/hep.29732.

16. Ambade A, Catalano D, Lim A, Kopoyan A, Shaffer SA, Mandrekar P. Inhibition of heat shock protein 90 alleviates steatosis and macrophage activation in murine alcoholic liver injury. J Hepatol. 2014;61:903–11. https://doi.org/10.1016/j.jhep.2014.05.024.
17. Saha B, Momen-Heravi F, Kodys K, Szabo G. MicroRNA cargo of extracellular vesicles from alcohol-exposed monocytes signals naive monocytes to differentiate into M2 macrophages. J Biol Chem. 2016;291:149–59. https://doi.org/10.1074/jbc.M115.694133.
18. Eguchi A, Wree A, Feldstein AE. Biomarkers of liver cell death. J Hepatol. 2014;60:1063–74. https://doi.org/10.1016/j.jhep.2013.12.026.
19. Momen-Heravi F, Saha B, Kodys K, Catalano D, Satishchandran A, Szabo G. Increased number of circulating exosomes and their microRNA cargos are potential novel biomarkers in alcoholic hepatitis. J Transl Med. 2015;13:261. https://doi.org/10.1186/s12967-015-0623-9.
20. Povero D, Eguchi A, Li H, Johnson CD, Papouchado BG, Wree A, Messer K, Feldstein AE. Circulating extracellular vesicles with specific proteome and liver microRNAs are potential biomarkers for liver injury in experimental fatty liver disease. PLoS One. 2014;9:e113651. https://doi.org/10.1371/journal.pone.0113651.
21. Garcia-Martinez I, Santoro N, Chen Y, Hoque R, Ouyang X, Caprio S, Shlomchik MJ, Coffman RL, Candia A, Mehal WZ. Hepatocyte mitochondrial DNA drives nonalcoholic steatohepatitis by activation of TLR9. J Clin Invest. 2016;126:859–64. https://doi.org/10.1172/JCI83885.
22. Povero D, Eguchi A, Niesman IR, Andronikou N, de Mollerat du Jeu X, Mulya A, Berk M, Lazic M, Thapaliya S, Parola M, et al. Lipid-induced toxicity stimulates hepatocytes to release angiogenic microparticles that require Vanin-1 for uptake by endothelial cells. Sci Signal. 2013;6:ra88. https://doi.org/10.1126/scisignal.2004512.

Chapter 7
Diabetes in Liver Disease

Takumi Kawaguchi, Dan Nakano, and Takuji Torimura

Abstract A high prevalence of diabetes mellitus has been reported in patients with chronic liver disease (CLD). Increasing evidence suggests that diabetes mellitus and its treatment have a significant impact on the clinical course of CLD. This review summarized the prevalence, diagnosis, and mechanisms of diabetes mellitus in patients with CLD. We also reviewed the clinical impact and therapeutic strategy for diabetes mellitus in patients with CLD. Recent progress using antidiabetic medication in non-alcoholic fatty liver disease/non-alcoholic steatohepatitis and hepatocellular carcinoma was also discussed.

Keywords Insulin resistance · Hepatitis C virus · Non-alcoholic fatty liver disease Steatohepatitis · Hepatoma · Dipeptidyl peptidase-4inhibitor · Sodium glucose cotransporter 2 inhibitor

Abbreviations

AMPK	AMP-activated kinase
CGMS	continuous glucose monitoring system
CI	confidence interval
CLD	chronic liver disease
DPP4	dipeptidyl peptidase IV
HbA1c	glycated hemoglobin
HBV	hepatitis B virus
HCC	hepatocellular carcinoma
HCV	hepatitis C virus
HR	hazard ratio
IGF-1	insulin-like growth factor-1

T. Kawaguchi (✉) · D. Nakano · T. Torimura
Division of Gastroenterology, Department of Medicine, Kurume University School of Medicine, Kurume, Japan
e-mail: takumi@med.kurume-u.ac.jp

H. Yoshiji, K. Kaji (eds.), *Alcoholic/Non-Alcoholic Digestive Diseases*,
https://doi.org/10.1007/978-981-13-1465-0_7

IGT	impaired glucose tolerance
Loxl2	lysyl oxidase like 2
MAPK	mitogen-activated protein kinase
NAFLD	non-alcoholic fatty liver disease
OR	odds ratio
PNPLA3	patatin-like phospholipase domain-containing 3
QOL	quality of life
SGLT2	sodium glucose cotransporter 2
VLDL	very-low-density lipoprotein

7.1 Prevalence of Impaired Glucose Tolerance (IGT) and Diabetes Mellitus in Patients with Chronic Liver Disease (CLD)

In 1967, Megyesi et al. reported that 32% of 28 patients with CLD had diabetes mellitus and 25% had IGT [1]. The features of diabetes mellitus in patients with CLD include insulin resistance and subsequent hyperinsulinemia, and diabetes mellitus that develops secondary to cirrhosis is called "hepatogenous diabetes" [1]. The prevalence of diabetes mellitus varies from 17.5 to 64.5% in patients with liver cirrhosis [2–4]. Nishida performed a systematic review on the prevalence of IGT and diabetes mellitus in patients with CLD and showed that of a total of 1747 patients with liver cirrhosis in 12 studies, 35.1% had diabetes mellitus and 27.8% had ITG [5]. Thus, more than 50% of patients with liver cirrhosis had IGT or diabetes mellitus (Fig. 7.1).

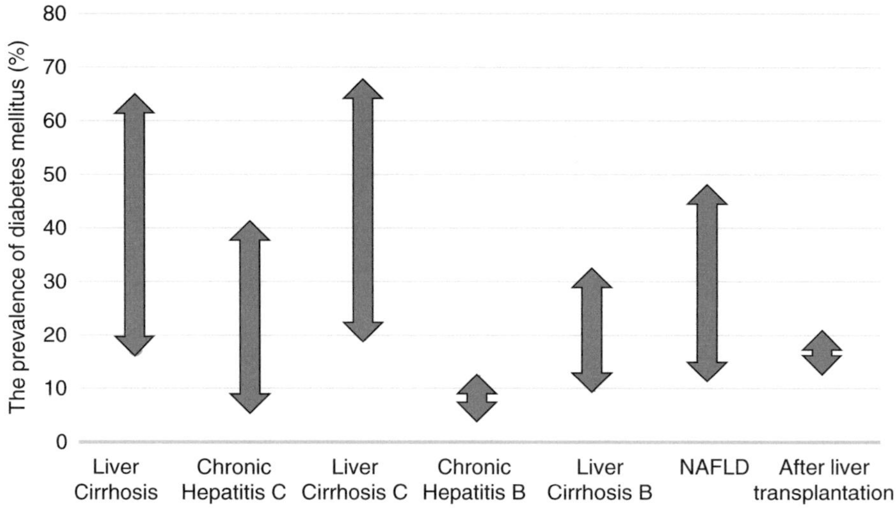

Fig. 7.1 Difference in the prevalence of diabetes mellitus in patients with chronic liver disease according to its etiology and severity of liver disease

7.1.1 Viral Hepatitis

Alavian et al. reported that diabetes mellitus was seen in 53.7% of patients with cirrhosis, 13.7% of those with chronic hepatitis, and 9.5% of hepatitis B virus (HBV) inactive carriers [6]. The prevalence of diabetes mellitus varies from 5.9 to 67.4% in patients with hepatitis C virus (HCV)-related liver disease [7–11], and from 4.3 to 31.6% in patients with HBV-related liver disease [9, 10, 12, 13] (Fig. 7.1). Fabiani et al. performed a meta-analysis of diabetes mellitus in patients with chronic HCV infection and reported its prevalence in 28.1% of those with cirrhosis and 17.2% of those with chronic hepatitis C [7]. They also investigated diabetes mellitus in patients with chronic HBV infection and demonstrated its prevalence in 13.7% of those with cirrhosis and 7.6% of those with chronic hepatitis B [7]. Thus, a higher prevalence of diabetes mellitus is seen in patients with HCV-related liver disease than in those with HBV-related liver disease (Fig. 7.1).

7.1.2 Non-alcoholic Fatty Liver Disease (NAFLD)

Ortiz-Lopez et al. demonstrated that 75% of patients with NAFLD have prediabetes and 14% have diabetes mellitus [14]. Imamura et al. also reported that the prevalence of diabetes mellitus increased significantly over a 20-year period among both men (6.0% in 1991 and 12.0% in 2011) and women (3.3% in 1991 and 5.1% in 2011) [15]. The prevalence of diabetes mellitus according to fibrosis stage (Stage 0/1/2/3/4) is 23.7/32.8/53.7/65.8 (%) in males and 34.7/45.2/60.9/64.7 (%) in females, respectively [16].

Newton et al. investigated type 2 diabetes mellitus in 675 children with NAFLD in a multicenter, cross-sectional study and showed a prediabetes prevalence of 23.4% and a diabetes mellitus prevalence of 6.5% [17]. Thus, a high prevalence of diabetes mellitus and IGT is seen in patients with NAFLD. In addition, about 30% of children with NAFLD also had prediabetes or diabetes mellitus.

7.1.3 New-Onset Diabetes Mellitus After Liver Transplantation

Diabetes mellitus frequently develops after liver transplantation. The incidence of new-onset diabetes mellitus after transplantation is 10.3–20.0% [18–23] (Fig. 7.1). Risk factors for post-transplant diabetes mellitus are male sex, pre-transplant diabetes mellitus, HCV infection, alcohol abuse, mycophenolate mofetil, and steroid pulse therapy for acute rejection [19, 21–23]. The prevalence of post-transplant diabetes mellitus has decreased with reduction in daily prednisone dose [24].

7.2 Diagnosis of Diabetes Mellitus in Patients with Liver Disease

7.2.1 Glycated Hemoglobin (HbA1c)

Measurement of HbA1c is used in the routine evaluation and management of patients with diabetes mellitus [25–27]. However, anemia due to hypersplenism is frequently seen in patients with liver cirrhosis and HbA1c in patients with liver cirrhosis was lower than that in patients with chronic hepatitis and diabetes mellitus in spite of equivalent glucose intolerance [28]. Other studies also demonstrated that HbA1c is not a reliable predictor of glycemic control in patients with liver cirrhosis [29, 30], and oral glucose tolerance testing, therefore, is recommended for the diagnosis of diabetes mellitus in patients with liver cirrhosis [28].

7.2.2 Continuous Glucose Monitoring System (CGMS)

A CGMS can assess 24-h glucose fluctuations and is useful for the detection of unnoticed hypo/hyperglycemic episodes [31, 32]. Isoda et al. examined glucose metabolism in 30 patients with liver cirrhosis using CGMS [33]. Although three patients had fasting glucose level > 126 mg/dL, 19 had average blood glucose level > 126 mg/dL, indicating that CGMS is a sensitive tool for detecting glucose disorders in patients with liver cirrhosis [33].

CGMS is also useful for evaluation of features of glucose abnormalities. Ochi et al. investigated the features of glucose abnormalities in patients with HCV infection and NAFLD [34]. They found that in patients with NAFLD, maximum blood glucose concentration is significantly correlated with hepatic fibrosis. In contrast, in patients with HCV-related liver disease, maximum blood glucose concentration is negatively correlated with serum albumin concentration [34]. Thus, hyperglycemia and excessive glycemic variability gradually progress in accordance with the progression of hepatic fibrosis from the early stage of CLD in patients with NAFLD. On the other hand, in patients with HCV-related liver disease, hyperglycemia and glycemic variability rapidly progress when hypoalbuminemia appears [34].

7.3 Mechanism of HCV- and NAFLD-Related Insulin Resistance

7.3.1 HCV-Related Insulin Resistance

High prevalence of diabetes mellitus is seen in patients with HCV-related liver disease [35–40]. In addition to inducing hepatic inflammation, HCV directly induces insulin resistance through various mechanisms. HCV downregulates insulin receptor substrates 1 and 2, which are central molecules involved in intracellular insulin signaling, by disturbing tyrosine phosphorylation or through upregulation of suppressor of cytokine signaling 3 [35, 41–44]. HCV infection also induces endoplasmic reticulum stress [44] and activation of mammalian target of rapamycin [45] and phosphatase 2A [46], leading to downregulation of insulin receptor substrates Akt and AMP-activated kinase (AMPK) [47, 48]. Moreover, HCV suppresses expression of glucose transporter 1 and 2 [49, 50] and downregulates glucagon-like peptide-1 in the gut through upregulation of dipeptidyl peptidase IV (DPP4), leading to an increase in blood glucose level [51].

HCV directly affects lipid metabolism, resulting in the development of insulin resistance. HCV core reduces microsomal triglyceride transfer protein function and decreases hepatic triglyceride secretion and assembly of very-low-density lipoprotein (VLDL) particles [52]. In addition, HCV induces miR-27, which downregulates peroxisome proliferator-activated receptor-α and angiopoietin-like protein 3, causing hepatic steatosis [53]. Moreover, HCV upregulates transcriptional activity of liver X receptor α, causing hepatic steatosis through increased expression of sterol regulatory element binding protein-1c, peroxisome proliferator-activated receptor-γ, and fatty acid synthase [54]. HCV also associates with VLDL components and forms lipoviral particles. HCV-lipoviral particles inhibit lipoprotein lipase activity, thereby inhibiting hydrolysis of triglyceride during the catabolic conversion of VLDL to low density lipoprotein [55].

Direct involvement of HCV in the development of insulin resistance can be confirmed by changes in glucose metabolism after treatment of HCV. After interferon-based treatment, there were no significant changes in insulin resistance in non-responders and relapsers; however, in sustained responders, insulin resistance was significantly decreased after interferon-based antiviral therapy [56]. HCV clearance by direct-acting antiviral treatments also reverses insulin resistance in chronic hepatitis C patients [57, 58].

7.3.2 NAFLD-Related Insulin Resistance

Although the pathogenesis of NAFLD remains unclear, a "multiple parallel hits hypothesis" has been proposed [59]. In patients with NAFLD, gut, adipose tissue, liver, and skeletal muscle are associated with the development of insulin resistance through the following mechanisms. (1) Intake of a fat-, fructose-, and cholesterol-rich diet causes a significant loss of tight junction proteins, leading to leaky gut and an increase in portal endotoxin levels [60, 61]. Changes in gut microbiota influence absorption and disposal of nutrients to the liver as well as hepatic inflammation by toll-like receptor ligands, leading to production of proinflammatory cytokines from hepatocytes [62]. (2) Fat accumulation in adipose tissue affects changes in adipokines including an increase in leptin, resistin, retinol binding protein-4, and chemerin and a decrease in adiponectin, omentin, and vaspin [63–66]. (3) Fat accumulation in hepatocytes causes not only hepatic inflammation, but also changes in hepatokines, including an increase in fetuin A, fetuin B, and selenoprotein P [67–70]. (4) Loss of skeletal muscle mass, sarcopenia, is involved in the development of insulin resistance in patients with NAFLD [71]. Serum irisin level, a myokine, is decreased in patients with NAFLD [72].

Genetic polymorphism is also associated with the development of NAFLD. Genetic polymorphisms are seen in patatin-like phospholipase domain-containing 3 (PNPLA3) [73, 74], neurocan [75], glucokinase regulatory protein [76], transmembrane 6-superfamily member 2 [77], and protein phosphatase 1 regulatory subunit 3B [78]. Among these genetic polymorphisms, a variant (rs738409 C > G p.I148M) in the *PNPLA3* gene is well documented [79]. PNPLA3 protein is located in lipid droplets in hepatocytes and hepatic stellate cells, and exerts hydrolase activity on triglycerides in hepatocytes and retinyl esters in hepatic stellate cells [79, 80]. The I148M mutation results in loss of function of the protein with fat accumulation in hepatocytes and retinol retention in hepatic stellate cells [79, 81, 82].

7.4 Clinical Impact

Diabetes mellitus is a risk factor for cardiovascular disease [83, 84]. In addition, diabetes mellitus is a risk factor for life-threatening complications including advanced hepatic fibrosis and hepatocellular carcinoma (HCC) in patients with either chronic HCV infection or NAFLD [85–88]. Moreover, diabetes mellitus impairs prognosis [89, 90] and quality of life (QOL) in patients with CLD [71, 91] (Table 7.1).

7.4.1 Hepatic Fibrosis and Gastroesophageal Varices

Diabetes and insulin resistance are risk factors for severe hepatic fibrosis in patients with chronic HCV infection and NAFLD [92, 93], and cirrhotic patients with diabetes mellitus have a higher risk of decompensation events [87]. In addition, diabetes mellitus is associated with gastroesophageal variceal bleeding in cirrhotic patients [94]. Insulin accelerates proliferation of hepatic stellate cells [95]; therefore, hyperinsulinemia is associated with advanced hepatic fibrosis [96, 97]. Several

Table 7.1 Clinical impact of diabetes mellitus in patients with chronic liver disease

Progression of hepatic fibrosis
Gastroesophageal variceal bleeding
Hepatic encephalopathy
Infection including spontaneous bacterial peritonitis
Sarcopenia
Hepatocarcinogenesis
Growth of hepatocellular carcinoma
Cardiovascular diseases
High mortality

mechanisms of insulin-induced activation of hepatic stellate cells have been reported. (1) Insulin upregulates connective tissue growth factor and type1 procollagen mRNA [98]; (2) insulin activates the PI3K/Akt-p70S6K pathway, which plays an important role in the early activation of hepatic stellate cells [99]; and (3) insulin upregulates metastasis-associated lung adenocarcinoma transcript 1 [100], which regulates Rac1 expression through miR-101b as a competing endogenous RNA, influencing the proliferation of hepatic stellate cells [101]. Furthermore, Dongiovanni et al. reported that hepatic expression of lysyl oxidase like 2 (Loxl2) is upregulated in NAFLD patients with diabetes mellitus, and hepatic and circulating Loxl2 levels are correlated with histological fibrosis progression [102]. Since Loxl2 is known to cross-link collagen and elastin in the extracellular matrix [103], Loxl2 may also be involved in the development of diabetes mellitus-induced hepatic fibrosis.

7.4.2 Hepatic Encephalopathy

Patients diagnosed with both compensated cirrhosis and diabetes mellitus have a higher risk of the development of decompensation events [87]. Diabetes mellitus increases the risk of first-time overt hepatic encephalopathy in cirrhotic patients [91]. A possible reason is that diabetes mellitus impairs hepatic encephalopathy by increasing glutaminase activity, impairing gut motility, and promoting constipation [104]. In addition, Bajaj et al. showed an increased relative abundance of Bacteroidaceae, Veillonellaceae, Streptococcaceae, and Eubacteriaceae, with a decrease in autochthonous Ruminococcaceae in cirrhotic patients with diabetes mellitus, suggesting that diabetes mellitus in the presence of cirrhosis alters the mucosal and stool microbiota [105].

7.4.3 Infection

Diabetes mellitus is a risk factor for infection and diabetes mellitus identified by oral glucose tolerance testing was significantly associated with a higher prevalence of infectious complications and death in a 3-month period in patients with liver cirrhosis [2]. Wlazlo et al. also reported that the presence of diabetes mellitus is associated with an increased risk of spontaneous bacterial peritonitis in patients with cirrhosis [106].

7.4.4 Sarcopenia

Sarcopenia is defined as a loss of skeletal muscle mass, strength, and function [107, 108]. Sarcopenia is a novel prognostic factor in patients with CLD [71, 109–113] and the Japan Society of Hepatology established new assessment criteria for sarcopenia in liver disease in 2015 [114]. Both CLD and diabetes mellitus are risk factors for sarcopenia [115, 116]. Recently, Hashimoto et al. demonstrated that skeletal muscle mass is negatively associated with NAFLD in men with diabetes mellitus [117]. However, limited information is available for the impact of diabetes mellitus on sarcopenia in patients with CLD including NAFLD.

7.4.5 HCC

Diabetes mellitus is an independent risk factor for HCC in patients with chronic HCV infection and NAFLD [88, 118–124]. Diabetes mellitus significantly increased the risk for HCC in hepatitis C patients aged 40–59 years old (hazard ratio [HR] 3.086; 95% confidence interval [CI]1.045–9.112) and in patients with NAFLD (HR 3.21; 95% CI 1.09–9.50) [125]. Insulin is a growth promoting hormone [126, 127] and hyperinsulinemia is associated with accelerated HCC growth in patients with CLD [128]. The following are possible mechanisms of insulin-induced HCC growth. (1) Insulin binds to insulin receptors and exerts mitogenic and cell proliferative effects through activation of the mitogen-activated protein kinase (MAPK)/extracellular signal-regulated kinase pathway [129, 130]. (2) Insulin also binds to insulin-like growth factor-1 (IGF-1) receptor and activates the Raf/MAPK kinase/MAPK cascade [131]. (3) Insulin binds to IGF-binding proteins, leading to an increase in serum free IGF-1 [132–135]. Thus, insulin resistance/hyperinsulinemia enhances hepatocarcinogenesis through multiple pathways.

7.4.6 Cardiovascular Disease

The prevalence of cardiovascular disease has been reported to be relatively low in cirrhotic patients with diabetes mellitus [136–138]. Lower coagulability and lipoprotein (a) level are thought to account for the low prevalence of microvascular disease in cirrhotic patients with diabetes mellitus [136, 137]. However, recent studies reported that diabetes mellitus increases cardiovascular disease in patients with chronic HCV infection and NAFLD [139–141]. Diabetes increases serum levels of platelet-derived apoptotic microparticles in patients with HCV infection, leading to the increased atherogenic risk associated with diabetes [139]. On the other hand, NAFLD was recently reported to be associated with an increased risk of developing microvascular diabetic complications including cardiovascular disease and chronic kidney disease [142–145]. Dallio et al. reported that endocan, an early marker of endothelial dysfunction, is elevated in patients with NAFLD [146]. Thus, diabetes mellitus and NAFLD synergistically increase cardiovascular disease [141].

7.4.7 *Mortality*

Diabetes mellitus increases risk of mortality in patients with CLD [89]. Diabetes mellitus is associated with an increased risk of both viral (HR 2.20; 95% CI 1.18–4.11) and non-viral hepatitis-related cirrhosis mortality (HR 3.06; 95% CI 2.13–4.41), and the association between diabetes mellitus and non-viral hepatitis-related cirrhosis mortality is stronger among patients with BMI <23 than in heavier individuals (HR 2.28; 95% CI 1.20–4.35) in Asia [147]. HCC is a leading causative factor of mortality and diabetes mellitus is independently associated with both poorer disease-free survival and poorer overall survival in HCC patients [86, 90, 148–150]. Recently, Huang et al. performed a multi-state model analysis to investigate transitions from "start-to-death" and "HCC-to-death" using the Taiwanese National Health Insurance Research Database [151]. They demonstrated that diabetes mellitus significantly increased the risk for transition from "start-to-death" (adjusted HR 2.61; 95% CI 2.05–3.33) and "HCC-to-death" (adjusted HR 1.36; 95% CI 1.10–1.68) [151]. Moreover, Younossi et al. reported that the presence of diabetes mellitus not only pre- and posttransplant in recipients, but also in donors is associated with an increased risk of adverse posttransplant outcomes [152].

7.5 Treatment

Nutritional therapy and exercise are first-line measures for diabetes mellitus, even in patients with CLD [126, 153, 154]. According to the guidelines on nutritional management in Japanese patients with liver cirrhosis aimed at preventing HCC, the standard for dietary intake is 25 kcal/kg (ideal body weight) per day, with protein intake of 1.0–1.5 g/kg/day and a 20–25% lipid:energy ratio [153]. For patients with NAFLD, both aerobic and resistance exercise reduce hepatic steatosis, based on similar frequency, duration, and period of exercise (40–45 min/session, 3 times/week for 12 weeks) [154].

There is no uniform strategy for pharmacotherapy of diabetes mellitus in patients with CLD [37, 38, 155]. However, insulin secretion is preserved in cirrhotic patients with diabetes mellitus [35, 156]. In addition, exogenous insulin and insulin secretagogues such as sulfonylureas are reported to increase the risk of HCC in patients with CLD [127, 157–160] (Table 7.2). On the other hand, insulin sensitizers such as metformin or thiazolidinediones are reported to reduce HCC risk in diabetic patients with CLD [157, 159–164] (Table 7.2). These insulin sensitizers exert antitumor effects by improving hyperinsulinemia as well as activation of AMPK and peroxisome proliferator-activated receptor γ [165, 166]. However, these medications are not always available for patients with advanced liver cirrhosis because of severe side effects. In addition, metformin was recently reported to increase tumor aggressiveness, and resistance to sorafenib caused upregulation of sirtuin-3 [167, 168] (Table 7.2).

Table 7.2 Effects of anti-diabetic agents on HCC

Anti-diabetic agent	Acceleration of HCC	Suppression of HCC
Exogenous insulin and sulfonylurea	[127, 157–160, 201–203]	
Metformin	[167, 168]	[157, 159–161, 163, 164, 203–207]
Thiazolidinediones		[160, 162]
DPP4 inhibitor	[180, 181][a]	
SGLT2 inhibitor		[198, 199][a]

[a]Data based on basic studies

7.5.1 Dipeptidyl Peptidase-4 (DPP-4) Inhibitor

DPP-4 inhibitor is effective and the most frequently prescribed antidiabetic medication in patients with CLD [158, 169–173]. In addition to inducing upregulation of glucagon-like peptide-1, DPP4 inhibitor has various other biological activities [174]. DPP4 inhibitor was reported to improve steatohepatitis in several animal models by downregulation of inflammatory genes (tumor necrosis factor-α, interleukin-6, and monocyte chemoattractant protein-1), suppressor of cytokine signaling 3, endoplasmic reticulum stress, and leukocyte cell-derived chemotaxin 2, and upregulation of AMPK [175–179]. On the other hand, DPP4 inhibitor is reported to upregulate metastatic capacity of HCC by activating nuclear factor E2-related factor 2 to decrease reactive oxygen species levels [180]. Harada et al. reported an association between DPP-4 inhibitor and rapid progression of HCC [181]. Thus, further study is required to evaluate beneficial effects of DPP4 inhibitor on patients with HCC.

7.5.2 SGLT2 Inhibitor

SGLT2 inhibitor blocks the reabsorption of filtered glucose in kidneys, resulting in improvement of hyperglycemia and subsequent hyperinsulinemia [182–184]. Beneficial effects of SGLT2 inhibitor on NAFLD have been reported in both basic and clinical studies [175, 185–194]. In addition, SGLT2 is reported to be present in pancreatic adenocarcinomas and SGLT2 inhibitor reduces tumor growth and survival in a xenograft model of pancreatic cancer [195]. SGLT2 is also present in colon cancer cells and exerts antitumor effects in colon cancer [196, 197]. Similarly, Obara et al. reported that SGLT2 inhibitor suppresses diethylnitrosamine-induced HCC tumorigenesis in obese and diabetic mice [198]. Kaji et al. also reported that SGLT2 inhibitor attenuates HCC growth and angiogenic activity by inhibiting glucose uptake in an animal model of HCC [199]. Recently, Tang et al. performed a systematic review of the association between SGLT2 inhibitors and risk of cancer in type 2 diabetes and found that SGLT2 inhibitors were not significantly associated with an overall increased risk of cancer [200]. In prespecified analysis, the risk of bladder cancer is increased with SGLT2 inhibitors (odds ratio [OR] 3.87; 95% CI 1.48–10.08); however, an SGLT2 inhibitor, canagliflozin, may have a preventive effect on gastrointestinal cancers (OR 0.15; 95% CI 0.04–0.60) [200]. As previous studies indicated antitumor effects of SGLT2 inhibitors, a large-scale, randomized control trial is required.

7.6 Conclusion

The prevalence of diabetes mellitus is high in patients with CLD. Diabetes mellitus is a risk factor for life-threatening complications, poor prognosis, and decreased QOL in patients with CLD. Recent studies suggest that insulin sensitizers such as metformin or thiazolidinediones, DPP4 inhibitors, and SGLT2 inhibitors have beneficial effects on liver disease. Therefore, treatment of diabetes mellitus may improve prognosis and QOL in patients with CLD.

Conflict of Interest Statement All authors disclose no conflicts.

Financial Support This work was supported by JSPS Grant-in-Aid for Scientific Research (C) JP17K09444.

References

1. Megyesi C, Samols E, Marks V. Glucose tolerance and diabetes in chronic liver disease. Lancet. 1967;2:1051–6.
2. Braganca AC, Alvares-da-Silva MR. Prevalence of diabetes mellitus and impaired glucose tolerance in patients with decompensated cirrhosis being evaluated for liver transplantation: the utility of oral glucose tolerance test. Arq Gastroenterol. 2010;47:22–7.
3. Jeon HK, Kim MY, Baik SK, Park HJ, Choi H, Park SY, et al. Hepatogenous diabetes in cirrhosis is related to portal pressure and variceal hemorrhage. Dig Dis Sci. 2013;58:3335–41.
4. Garcia-Compean D, Jaquez-Quintana JO, Lavalle-Gonzalez FJ, Gonzalez-Gonzalez JA, Munoz-Espinosa LE, Villarreal-Perez JZ, et al. Subclinical abnormal glucose tolerance is a predictor of death in liver cirrhosis. World J Gastroenterol. 2014;20:7011–8.
5. Nishida T. Diagnosis and clinical implications of diabetes in liver cirrhosis: a focus on the oral glucose tolerance test. J Endocr Soc. 2017;1:886–96.
6. Alavian SM, Hajarizadeh B, Nematizadeh F, Larijani B. Prevalence and determinants of diabetes mellitus among Iranian patients with chronic liver disease. BMC Endocr Disord. 2004;4:4.
7. Fabiani S, Fallahi P, Ferrari SM, Miccoli M, Antonelli A. Hepatitis C virus infection and development of type 2 diabetes mellitus: systematic review and meta-analysis of the literature. Rev Endocr Metab Disord. 2018;19(4):405–20.
8. Thuluvath PJ, John PR. Association between hepatitis C, diabetes mellitus, and race. A case-control study. Am J Gastroenterol. 2003;98:438–41.
9. Rouabhia S, Malek R, Bounecer H, Dekaken A, Bendali Amor F, Sadelaoud M, et al. Prevalence of type 2 diabetes in Algerian patients with hepatitis C virus infection. World J Gastroenterol. 2010;16:3427–31.

10. Mangia A, Schiavone G, Lezzi G, Marmo R, Bruno F, Villani MR, et al. HCV and diabetes mellitus: evidence for a negative association. Am J Gastroenterol. 1998;93:2363–7.
11. Labropoulou-Karatza C, Goritsas C, Fragopanagou H, Repandi M, Matsouka P, Alexandrides T. High prevalence of diabetes mellitus among adult beta-thalassaemic patients with chronic hepatitis C. Eur J Gastroenterol Hepatol. 1999;11:1033–6.
12. Knobler H, Schihmanter R, Zifroni A, Fenakel G, Schattner A. Increased risk of type 2 diabetes in noncirrhotic patients with chronic hepatitis C virus infection. Mayo Clin Proc. 2000;75:355–9.
13. Caronia S, Taylor K, Pagliaro L, Carr C, Palazzo U, Petrik J, et al. Further evidence for an association between non-insulin-dependent diabetes mellitus and chronic hepatitis C virus infection. Hepatology. 1999;30:1059–63.
14. Ortiz-Lopez C, Lomonaco R, Orsak B, Finch J, Chang Z, Kochunov VG, et al. Prevalence of prediabetes and diabetes and metabolic profile of patients with nonalcoholic fatty liver disease (NAFLD). Diabetes Care. 2012;35:873–8.
15. Imamura Y, Uto H, Hiramine Y, Hosoyamada K, Ijuin S, Yoshifuku S, et al. Increasing prevalence of diabetes mellitus in association with fatty liver in a Japanese population. J Gastroenterol. 2014;49:1406–13.
16. Nakahara T, Hyogo H, Yoneda M, Sumida Y, Eguchi Y, Fujii H, et al. Type 2 diabetes mellitus is associated with the fibrosis severity in patients with nonalcoholic fatty liver disease in a large retrospective cohort of Japanese patients. J Gastroenterol. 2014;49:1477–84.
17. Newton KP, Hou J, Crimmins NA, Lavine JE, Barlow SE, Xanthakos SA, et al. Prevalence of prediabetes and type 2 diabetes in children with nonalcoholic fatty liver disease. JAMA Pediatr. 2016;170:e161971.
18. Cho JM, Oh SH, Kim KM, Namgung JM, Kim DY, Song GW, et al. Prevalence and treatment of new-onset diabetes mellitus after liver transplantation in Korean children: a single-center study. Transplant Proc. 2014;46:873–5.
19. Parolin MB, Zaina FE, Araujo MV, Kupka E, Coelho JC. Prevalence of new-onset diabetes mellitus in Brazilian liver transplant recipients: association with HCV infection. Transplant Proc. 2004;36:2776–7.
20. Saab S, Shpaner A, Zhao Y, Brito I, Durazo F, Han S, et al. Prevalence and risk factors for diabetes mellitus in moderate term survivors of liver transplantation. Am J Transplant. 2006;6:1890–5.
21. Honda M, Asonuma K, Hayashida S, Suda H, Ohya Y, Lee KJ, et al. Incidence and risk factors for new-onset diabetes in living-donor liver transplant recipients. Clin Transpl. 2013;27:426–35.
22. Anastacio LR, Ribeiro Hde S, Ferreira LG, Lima AS, Vilela EG, Toulson Davisson Correia MI. Incidence and risk factors for diabetes, hypertension and obesity after liver transplantation. Nutr Hosp. 2013;28:643–8.
23. Hara Y, Kawagishi N, Nakanishi W, Tokodai K, Nakanishi C, Miyagi S, et al. Prevalence and risk factors of obesity, hypertension, dyslipidemia and diabetes mellitus before and after adult living donor liver transplantation. Hepatol Res. 2015;45:764–70.
24. Navasa M, Bustamante J, Marroni C, Gonzalez E, Andreu H, Esmatjes E, et al. Diabetes mellitus after liver transplantation: prevalence and predictive factors. J Hepatol. 1996;25:64–71.
25. Chamberlain JJ, Herman WH, Leal S, Rhinehart AS, Shubrook JH, Skolnik N, et al. Pharmacologic therapy for type 2 diabetes: synopsis of the 2017 American Diabetes Association Standards of Medical Care in Diabetes. Ann Intern Med. 2017;166:572–8.
26. Trenti T, Cristani A, Cioni G, Pentore R, Mussini C, Ventura E. Fructosamine and glycated hemoglobin as indices of glycemic control in patients with liver cirrhosis. Ric Clin Lab. 1990;20:261–7.
27. Araki E, Haneda M, Kasuga M, Nishikawa T, Kondo T, Ueki K, et al. New glycemic targets for patients with diabetes from the Japan Diabetes Society. J Diabetes Investig. 2017;8:123–5.
28. Nomura Y, Nanjo K, Miyano M, Kikuoka H, Kuriyama S, Maeda M, et al. Hemoglobin A1 in cirrhosis of the liver. Diabetes Res. 1989;11:177–80.

29. Cacciatore L, Cozzolino G, Giardina MG, De Marco F, Sacca L, Esposito P, et al. Abnormalities of glucose metabolism induced by liver cirrhosis and glycosylated hemoglobin levels in chronic liver disease. Diabetes Res. 1988;7:185–8.
30. Nadelson J, Satapathy SK, Nair S. Glycated hemoglobin levels in patients with decompensated cirrhosis. Int J Endocrinol. 2016;2016:8390210.
31. Currie CJ, Poole CD, Papo NL. An overview and commentary on retrospective, continuous glucose monitoring for the optimisation of care for people with diabetes. Curr Med Res Opin. 2009;25:2389–400.
32. Kawaguchi T, Itou M, Taniguchi E, Sakata M, Abe M, Koga H, et al. Serum level of free fatty acids is associated with nocturnal hypoglycemia in cirrhotic patients with HCV infection: a pilot study. Hepatogastroenterology. 2011;58:103–8.
33. Isoda H, Takahashi H, Eguchi Y, Kojima M, Inoue K, Murayama K, et al. Re-evaluation of glycated hemoglobin and glycated albumin with continuous glucose monitoring system as markers of glycemia in patients with liver cirrhosis. Biomed Rep. 2017;6:51–6.
34. Ochi T, Kawaguchi T, Nakahara T, Ono M, Noguchi S, Koshiyama Y, et al. Differences in characteristics of glucose intolerance between patients with NAFLD and chronic hepatitis C as determined by CGMS. Sci Rep. 2017;7:10146.
35. Kawaguchi T, Yoshida T, Harada M, Hisamoto T, Nagao Y, Ide T, et al. Hepatitis C virus down-regulates insulin receptor substrates 1 and 2 through up-regulation of suppressor of cytokine signaling 3. Am J Pathol. 2004;165:1499–508.
36. Kawaguchi T, Nagao Y, Tanaka K, Ide T, Harada M, Kumashiro R, et al. Causal relationship between hepatitis C virus core and the development of type 2 diabetes mellitus in a hepatitis C virus hyperendemic area: a pilot study. Int J Mol Med. 2005;16:109–14.
37. Kawaguchi T, Sata M. Importance of hepatitis C virus-associated insulin resistance: therapeutic strategies for insulin sensitization. World J Gastroenterol. 2010;16:1943–52.
38. Kawaguchi T, Taniguchi E, Itou M, Sumie S, Yamagishi S, Sata M. The pathogenesis, complications and therapeutic strategy for hepatitis C virus-associated insulin resistance in the era of anti-viral treatment. Rev Recent Clin Trials. 2010;5:147–57.
39. Kawaguchi T, Taniguchi E, Itou M, Sakata M, Sumie S, Sata M. Insulin resistance and chronic liver disease. World J Hepatol. 2011;3:99–107.
40. Kawaguchi T, Sata M. Glucose metabolism disorder: a risk factor for hepatocellular carcinoma. Nihon Shokakibyo Gakkai Zasshi. 2012;109:544–54.
41. Shintani Y, Fujie H, Miyoshi H, Tsutsumi T, Tsukamoto K, Kimura S, et al. Hepatitis C virus infection and diabetes: direct involvement of the virus in the development of insulin resistance. Gastroenterology. 2004;126:840–8.
42. Pazienza V, Clement S, Pugnale P, Conzelman S, Foti M, Mangia A, et al. The hepatitis C virus core protein of genotypes 3a and 1b downregulates insulin receptor substrate 1 through genotype-specific mechanisms. Hepatology. 2007;45:1164–71.
43. Pascarella S, Clement S, Guilloux K, Conzelmann S, Penin F, Negro F. Effects of hepatitis C virus on suppressor of cytokine signaling mRNA levels: comparison between different genotypes and core protein sequence analysis. J Med Virol. 2011;83:1005–15.
44. Ahmed QL, Manzoor S, Tariq M, Khalid M, Ashraf W, Parvaiz F, et al. Hepatitis C virus infection in vitro triggers endoplasmic reticulum stress and downregulates insulin receptor substrates 1 and 2 through upregulation of cytokine signaling suppressor 3. Acta Virol. 2014;58:238–44.
45. Bose SK, Shrivastava S, Meyer K, Ray RB, Ray R. Hepatitis C virus activates the mTOR/S6K1 signaling pathway in inhibiting IRS-1 function for insulin resistance. J Virol. 2012;86:6315–22.
46. Bernsmeier C, Duong FH, Christen V, Pugnale P, Negro F, Terracciano L, et al. Virus-induced over-expression of protein phosphatase 2A inhibits insulin signalling in chronic hepatitis C. J Hepatol. 2008;49:429–40.
47. del Campo JA, Garcia-Valdecasas M, Rojas L, Rojas A, Romero-Gomez M. The hepatitis C virus modulates insulin signaling pathway in vitro promoting insulin resistance. PLoS One. 2012;7:e47904.

48. Gastaldi G, Goossens N, Clement S, Negro F. Current level of evidence on causal association between hepatitis C virus and type 2 diabetes: a review. J Adv Res. 2017;8:149–59.
49. Kasai D, Adachi T, Deng L, Nagano-Fujii M, Sada K, Ikeda M, et al. HCV replication suppresses cellular glucose uptake through down-regulation of cell surface expression of glucose transporters. J Hepatol. 2009;50:883–94.
50. Lerat H, Imache MR, Polyte J, Gaudin A, Mercey M, Donati F, et al. Hepatitis C virus induces a prediabetic state by directly impairing hepatic glucose metabolism in mice. J Biol Chem. 2017;292:12860–73.
51. Itou M, Kawaguchi T, Taniguchi E, Sumie S, Oriishi T, Mitsuyama K, et al. Altered expression of glucagon-like peptide-1 and dipeptidyl peptidase IV in patients with HCV-related glucose intolerance. J Gastroenterol Hepatol. 2008;23:244–51.
52. Yamaguchi A, Tazuma S, Nishioka T, Ohishi W, Hyogo H, Nomura S, et al. Hepatitis C virus core protein modulates fatty acid metabolism and thereby causes lipid accumulation in the liver. Dig Dis Sci. 2005;50:1361–71.
53. Singaravelu R, Chen R, Lyn RK, Jones DM, O'Hara S, Rouleau Y, et al. Hepatitis C virus induced up-regulation of microRNA-27: a novel mechanism for hepatic steatosis. Hepatology. 2014;59:98–108.
54. Garcia-Mediavilla MV, Pisonero-Vaquero S, Lima-Cabello E, Benedicto I, Majano PL, Jorquera F, et al. Liver X receptor alpha-mediated regulation of lipogenesis by core and NS5A proteins contributes to HCV-induced liver steatosis and HCV replication. Lab Invest. 2012;92:1191–202.
55. Sun HY, Lin CC, Lee JC, Wang SW, Cheng PN, Wu IC, et al. Very low-density lipoprotein/lipo-viro particles reverse lipoprotein lipase-mediated inhibition of hepatitis C virus infection via apolipoprotein C-III. Gut. 2013;62:1193–203.
56. Kawaguchi T, Ide T, Taniguchi E, Hirano E, Itou M, Sumie S, et al. Clearance of HCV improves insulin resistance, beta-cell function, and hepatic expression of insulin receptor substrate 1 and 2. Am J Gastroenterol. 2007;102:570–6.
57. Adinolfi LE, Nevola R, Guerrera B, D'Alterio G, Marrone A, Giordano M, et al. HCV clearance by direct-acting antiviral treatments reverses insulin resistance in chronic hepatitis C patients. J Gastroenterol Hepatol. 2018;33(7):1379–82.
58. Ciancio A, Bosio R, Bo S, Pellegrini M, Sacco M, Vogliotti E, et al. Significant improvement of glycemic control in diabetic patients with HCV infection responding to direct-acting antiviral agents. J Med Virol. 2018;90:320–7.
59. Tilg H, Moschen AR. Evolution of inflammation in nonalcoholic fatty liver disease: the multiple parallel hits hypothesis. Hepatology. 2010;52:1836–46.
60. Brandt A, Jin CJ, Nolte K, Sellmann C, Engstler AJ, Bergheim I. Short-term intake of a fructose-, fat- and cholesterol-rich diet causes hepatic steatosis in mice: effect of antibiotic treatment. Nutrients. 2017;9:E1013.
61. Imajo K, Fujita K, Yoneda M, Nozaki Y, Ogawa Y, Shinohara Y, et al. Hyperresponsivity to low-dose endotoxin during progression to nonalcoholic steatohepatitis is regulated by leptin-mediated signaling. Cell Metab. 2012;16:44–54.
62. Mencin A, Kluwe J, Schwabe RF. Toll-like receptors as targets in chronic liver diseases. Gut. 2009;58:704–20.
63. Polyzos SA, Kountouras J, Mantzoros CS. Adipokines in nonalcoholic fatty liver disease. Metabolism. 2016;65:1062–79.
64. Polyzos SA, Kountouras J, Polymerou V, Papadimitriou KG, Zavos C, Katsinelos P. Vaspin, resistin, retinol-binding protein-4, interleukin-1alpha and interleukin-6 in patients with nonalcoholic fatty liver disease. Ann Hepatol. 2016;15:705–14.
65. Zwolak A, Szuster-Ciesielska A, Daniluk J, Semeniuk J, Kandefer-Szerszen M. Chemerin, retinol binding protein-4, cytokeratin-18 and transgelin-2 presence in sera of patients with non-alcoholic liver fatty disease. Ann Hepatol. 2016;15:862–9.
66. Aktas B, Yilmaz Y, Eren F, Yonal O, Kurt R, Alahdab YO, et al. Serum levels of vaspin, obestatin, and apelin-36 in patients with nonalcoholic fatty liver disease. Metabolism. 2011;60:544–9.

67. Misu H, Takamura T, Takayama H, Hayashi H, Matsuzawa-Nagata N, Kurita S, et al. A liver-derived secretory protein, selenoprotein P, causes insulin resistance. Cell Metab. 2010;12:483–95.
68. von Loeffelholz C, Horn P, Birkenfeld AL, Claus RA, Metzing BU, Docke S, et al. Fetuin A is a predictor of liver fat in preoperative patients with nonalcoholic fatty liver disease. J Invest Surg. 2016;29:266–74.
69. Meex RCR, Watt MJ. Hepatokines: linking nonalcoholic fatty liver disease and insulin resistance. Nat Rev Endocrinol. 2017;13:509–20.
70. Ebert T, Linder N, Schaudinn A, Busse H, Berger J, Lichtinghagen R, et al. Association of fetuin B with markers of liver fibrosis in nonalcoholic fatty liver disease. Endocrine. 2017;58:246–52.
71. Bhanji RA, Narayanan P, Allen AM, Malhi H, Watt KD. Sarcopenia in hiding: the risk and consequence of underestimating muscle dysfunction in nonalcoholic steatohepatitis. Hepatology. 2017;66:2055–65.
72. Polyzos SA, Kountouras J, Anastasilakis AD, Geladari EV, Mantzoros CS. Irisin in patients with nonalcoholic fatty liver disease. Metabolism. 2014;63:207–17.
73. Kawaguchi T, Sumida Y, Umemura A, Matsuo K, Takahashi M, Takamura T, et al. Genetic polymorphisms of the human PNPLA3 gene are strongly associated with severity of non-alcoholic fatty liver disease in Japanese. PLoS One. 2012;7:e38322.
74. Romeo S, Kozlitina J, Xing C, Pertsemlidis A, Cox D, Pennacchio LA, et al. Genetic variation in PNPLA3 confers susceptibility to nonalcoholic fatty liver disease. Nat Genet. 2008;40:1461–5.
75. Palmer ND, Musani SK, Yerges-Armstrong LM, Feitosa MF, Bielak LF, Hernaez R, et al. Characterization of European ancestry nonalcoholic fatty liver disease-associated variants in individuals of African and Hispanic descent. Hepatology. 2013;58:966–75.
76. Hernaez R, McLean J, Lazo M, Brancati FL, Hirschhorn JN, Borecki IB, et al. Association between variants in or near PNPLA3, GCKR, and PPP1R3B with ultrasound-defined steatosis based on data from the third National Health and Nutrition Examination Survey. Clin Gastroenterol Hepatol. 2013;11:1183–1190e1182.
77. Sookoian S, Pirola CJ. Meta-analysis of the influence of TM6SF2 E167K variant on plasma concentration of aminotransferases across different populations and diverse liver phenotypes. Sci Rep. 2016;6:27718.
78. Speliotes EK, Yerges-Armstrong LM, Wu J, Hernaez R, Kim LJ, Palmer CD, et al. Genome-wide association analysis identifies variants associated with nonalcoholic fatty liver disease that have distinct effects on metabolic traits. PLoS Genet. 2011;7:e1001324.
79. Trepo E, Romeo S, Zucman-Rossi J, Nahon P. PNPLA3 gene in liver diseases. J Hepatol. 2016;65:399–412.
80. Pirazzi C, Valenti L, Motta BM, Pingitore P, Hedfalk K, Mancina RM, et al. PNPLA3 has retinyl-palmitate lipase activity in human hepatic stellate cells. Hum Mol Genet. 2014;23:4077–85.
81. He S, McPhaul C, Li JZ, Garuti R, Kinch L, Grishin NV, et al. A sequence variation (I148M) in PNPLA3 associated with nonalcoholic fatty liver disease disrupts triglyceride hydrolysis. J Biol Chem. 2010;285:6706–15.
82. Huang Y, Cohen JC, Hobbs HH. Expression and characterization of a PNPLA3 protein isoform (I148M) associated with nonalcoholic fatty liver disease. J Biol Chem. 2011;286:37085–93.
83. Nordt TK, Schneider DJ, Sobel BE. Augmentation of the synthesis of plasminogen activator inhibitor type-1 by precursors of insulin. A potential risk factor for vascular disease. Circulation. 1994;89:321–30.
84. Haffner SM, Howard G, Mayer E, Bergman RN, Savage PJ, Rewers M, et al. Insulin sensitivity and acute insulin response in African-Americans, non-Hispanic whites, and Hispanics with NIDDM: the insulin resistance atherosclerosis study. Diabetes. 1997;46:63–9.
85. Eslam M, Kawaguchi T, Del Campo JA, Sata M, Khattab MA, Romero-Gomez M. Use of HOMA-IR in hepatitis C. J Viral Hepat. 2011;18:675–84.

86. Farrell G. Insulin resistance, obesity, and liver cancer. Clin Gastroenterol Hepatol. 2014;12:117–9.
87. Liu TL, Trogdon J, Weinberger M, Fried B, Barritt AS. Diabetes is associated with clinical decompensation events in patients with cirrhosis. Dig Dis Sci. 2016;61:3335–45.
88. Yang JD, Mohamed HA, Cvinar JL, Gores GJ, Roberts LR, Kim WR. Diabetes mellitus heightens the risk of hepatocellular carcinoma except in patients with hepatitis C cirrhosis. Am J Gastroenterol. 2016;111:1573–80.
89. Wild SH, Morling JR, McAllister DA, Kerssens J, Fischbacher C, Parkes J, et al. Type 2 diabetes and risk of hospital admission or death for chronic liver diseases. J Hepatol. 2016;64:1358–64.
90. Su YW, Liu PH, Hsu CY, Lee YH, Hsia CY, Ho SY, et al. Prognostic impact of diabetes mellitus on hepatocellular carcinoma: special emphasis from the BCLC perspective. PLoS One. 2017;12:e0174333.
91. Jepsen P, Watson H, Andersen PK, Vilstrup H. Diabetes as a risk factor for hepatic encephalopathy in cirrhosis patients. J Hepatol. 2015;63:1133–8.
92. Fracanzani AL, Valenti L, Bugianesi E, Andreoletti M, Colli A, Vanni E, et al. Risk of severe liver disease in nonalcoholic fatty liver disease with normal aminotransferase levels: a role for insulin resistance and diabetes. Hepatology. 2008;48:792–8.
93. Patel S, Jinjuvadia R, Patel R, Liangpunsakul S. Insulin resistance is associated with significant liver fibrosis in chronic hepatitis C patients: a systemic review and meta-analysis. J Clin Gastroenterol. 2016;50:80–4.
94. Yang CH, Chiu YC, Chen CH, Chen CH, Tsai MC, Chuah SK, et al. Diabetes mellitus is associated with gastroesophageal variceal bleeding in cirrhotic patients. Kaohsiung J Med Sci. 2014;30:515–20.
95. Li Q, Li X, Deng CL. Induction of proliferation and activation of rat hepatic stellate cells via high glucose and high insulin. Eur Rev Med Pharmacol Sci. 2017;21:5420–9.
96. Ota T, Takamura T, Kurita S, Matsuzawa N, Kita Y, Uno M, et al. Insulin resistance accelerates a dietary rat model of nonalcoholic steatohepatitis. Gastroenterology. 2007;132:282–93.
97. Kaji K, Yoshiji H, Kitade M, Ikenaka Y, Noguchi R, Yoshii J, et al. Impact of insulin resistance on the progression of chronic liver diseases. Int J Mol Med. 2008;22:801–8.
98. Paradis V, Perlemuter G, Bonvoust F, Dargere D, Parfait B, Vidaud M, et al. High glucose and hyperinsulinemia stimulate connective tissue growth factor expression: a potential mechanism involved in progression to fibrosis in nonalcoholic steatohepatitis. Hepatology. 2001;34:738–44.
99. Cai CX, Buddha H, Castelino-Prabhu S, Zhang Z, Britton RS, Bacon BR, et al. Activation of insulin-PI3K/Akt-p70S6K pathway in hepatic stellate cells contributes to fibrosis in nonalcoholic steatohepatitis. Dig Dis Sci. 2017;62:968–78.
100. Leti F, Legendre C, Still CD, Chu X, Petrick A, Gerhard GS, et al. Altered expression of MALAT1 lncRNA in nonalcoholic steatohepatitis fibrosis regulates CXCL5 in hepatic stellate cells. Transl Res. 2017;190:25–39 e21.
101. Yu F, Lu Z, Cai J, Huang K, Chen B, Li G, et al. MALAT1 functions as a competing endogenous RNA to mediate Rac1 expression by sequestering miR-101b in liver fibrosis. Cell Cycle. 2015;14:3885–96.
102. Dongiovanni P, Meroni M, Baselli GA, Bassani GA, Rametta R, Pietrelli A, et al. Insulin resistance promotes Lysyl Oxidase Like 2 induction and fibrosis accumulation in nonalcoholic fatty liver disease. Clin Sci (Lond). 2017;131:1301–15.
103. Moon HJ, Finney J, Ronnebaum T, Mure M. Human lysyl oxidase-like 2. Bioorg Chem. 2014;57:231–41.
104. Ampuero J, Ranchal I, del Mar Diaz-Herrero M, del Campo JA, Bautista JD, Romero-Gomez M. Role of diabetes mellitus on hepatic encephalopathy. Metab Brain Dis. 2013;28:277–9.
105. Bajaj JS, Betrapally NS, Hylemon PB, Thacker LR, Daita K, Kang DJ, et al. Gut microbiota alterations can predict hospitalizations in cirrhosis independent of diabetes mellitus. Sci Rep. 2015;5:18559.

106. Wlazlo N, van Greevenbroek MM, Curvers J, Schoon EJ, Friederich P, Twisk JW, et al. Diabetes mellitus at the time of diagnosis of cirrhosis is associated with higher incidence of spontaneous bacterial peritonitis, but not with increased mortality. Clin Sci (Lond). 2013;125:341–8.
107. Chen LK, Liu LK, Woo J, Assantachai P, Auyeung TW, Bahyah KS, et al. Sarcopenia in Asia: consensus report of the Asian Working Group for Sarcopenia. J Am Med Dir Assoc. 2014;15:95–101.
108. Cruz-Jentoft AJ, Baeyens JP, Bauer JM, Boirie Y, Cederholm T, Landi F, et al. Sarcopenia: European consensus on definition and diagnosis: report of the European Working Group on Sarcopenia in older people. Age Ageing. 2010;39:412–23.
109. Iwasa M, Hara N, Terasaka E, Hattori A, Ishidome M, Mifuji-Moroka R, et al. Evaluation and prognosis of sarcopenia using impedance analysis in patients with liver cirrhosis. Hepatol Res. 2014;44:E316–7.
110. Hanai T, Shiraki M, Nishimura K, Ohnishi S, Imai K, Suetsugu A, et al. Sarcopenia impairs prognosis of patients with liver cirrhosis. Nutrition. 2015;31:193–9.
111. Fujiwara N, Nakagawa H, Kudo Y, Tateishi R, Taguri M, Watadani T, et al. Sarcopenia, intramuscular fat deposition, and visceral adiposity independently predict the outcomes of hepatocellular carcinoma. J Hepatol. 2015;63:131–40.
112. Imai K, Takai K, Watanabe S, Hanai T, Suetsugu A, Shiraki M, et al. Sarcopenia impairs prognosis of patients with hepatocellular carcinoma: the role of liver functional reserve and tumor-related factors in loss of skeletal muscle volume. Nutrients. 2017;9:E1054.
113. Kim G, Kang SH, Kim MY, Baik SK. Prognostic value of sarcopenia in patients with liver cirrhosis: a systematic review and meta-analysis. PLoS One. 2017;12:e0186990.
114. Nishikawa H, Shiraki M, Hiramatsu A, Moriya K, Hino K, Nishiguchi S. Japan Society of Hepatology guidelines for sarcopenia in liver disease (1st edition): recommendation from the working group for creation of sarcopenia assessment criteria. Hepatol Res. 2016;46:951–63.
115. Fukuda T, Bouchi R, Takeuchi T, Nakano Y, Murakami M, Minami I, et al. Association of diabetic retinopathy with both sarcopenia and muscle quality in patients with type 2 diabetes: a cross-sectional study. BMJ Open Diabetes Res Care. 2017;5:e000404.
116. Benjamin J, Shasthry V, Kaal CR, Anand L, Bhardwaj A, Pandit V, et al. Characterization of body composition and definition of sarcopenia in patients with alcoholic cirrhosis: a computed tomography based study. Liver Int. 2017;37:1668–74.
117. Hashimoto Y, Osaka T, Fukuda T, Tanaka M, Yamazaki M, Fukui M. The relationship between hepatic steatosis and skeletal muscle mass index in men with type 2 diabetes. Endocr J. 2016;63:877–84.
118. Abad IR. Descriptive study of cancer of the cavum, particularly epidermoid carcinoma (1). Acta Otorrinolaringol Esp. 1989;40:81–99.
119. Hassan MM, Hwang LY, Hatten CJ, Swaim M, Li D, Abbruzzese JL, et al. Risk factors for hepatocellular carcinoma: synergism of alcohol with viral hepatitis and diabetes mellitus. Hepatology. 2002;36:1206–13.
120. Davila JA, Morgan RO, Shaib Y, McGlynn KA, El-Serag HB. Diabetes increases the risk of hepatocellular carcinoma in the United States: a population based case control study. Gut. 2005;54:533–9.
121. Dyal HK, Aguilar M, Bartos G, Holt EW, Bhuket T, Liu B, et al. Diabetes mellitus increases risk of hepatocellular carcinoma in chronic hepatitis C virus patients: a systematic review. Dig Dis Sci. 2016;61:636–45.
122. Reeves HL, Zaki MY, Day CP. Hepatocellular carcinoma in obesity, type 2 diabetes, and NAFLD. Dig Dis Sci. 2016;61:1234–45.
123. Mantovani A, Targher G. Type 2 diabetes mellitus and risk of hepatocellular carcinoma: spotlight on nonalcoholic fatty liver disease. Ann Transl Med. 2017;5:270.
124. Simon TG, King LY, Chong DQ, Nguyen L, Ma Y, VoPham T, et al. Diabetes, metabolic comorbidities and risk of hepatocellular carcinoma: results from two prospective cohort studies. Hepatology. 2018;67(5):1797–806.

125. Huang YW, Wang TC, Yang SS, Lin SY, Fu SC, Hu JT, et al. Increased risk of hepatocellular carcinoma in chronic hepatitis C patients with new onset diabetes: a nation-wide cohort study. Aliment Pharmacol Ther. 2015;42:902–11.
126. Kawaguchi T, Izumi N, Charlton MR, Sata M. Branched-chain amino acids as pharmacological nutrients in chronic liver disease. Hepatology. 2011;54:1063–70.
127. Sandow J. Growth effects of insulin and insulin analogues. Arch Physiol Biochem. 2009;115:72–85.
128. Saito K, Inoue S, Saito T, Kiso S, Ito N, Tamura S, et al. Augmentation effect of postprandial hyperinsulinaemia on growth of human hepatocellular carcinoma. Gut. 2002;51:100–4.
129. Barker BE, Fanger H, Farnes P. Human mammary slices in organ culture. I. Method of culture and preliminary observations on the effect of insulin. Exp Cell Res. 1964;35:437–48.
130. Formisano P, Oriente F, Fiory F, Caruso M, Miele C, Maitan MA, et al. Insulin-activated protein kinase Cbeta bypasses Ras and stimulates mitogen-activated protein kinase activity and cell proliferation in muscle cells. Mol Cell Biol. 2000;20:6323–33.
131. Sandhu MS, Dunger DB, Giovannucci EL. Insulin, insulin-like growth factor-I (IGF-I), IGF binding proteins, their biologic interactions, and colorectal cancer. J Natl Cancer Inst. 2002;94:972–80.
132. Le Roith D. Seminars in medicine of the Beth Israel Deaconess Medical Center. Insulin-like growth factors. N Engl J Med. 1997;336:633–40.
133. Scharf JG, Dombrowski F, Ramadori G. The IGF axis and hepatocarcinogenesis. Mol Pathol. 2001;54:138–44.
134. Alexia C, Fallot G, Lasfer M, Schweizer-Groyer G, Groyer A. An evaluation of the role of insulin-like growth factors (IGF) and of type-I IGF receptor signalling in hepatocarcinogenesis and in the resistance of hepatocarcinoma cells against drug-induced apoptosis. Biochem Pharmacol. 2004;68:1003–15.
135. Hung CH, Wang JH, Hu TH, Chen CH, Chang KC, Yen YH, et al. Insulin resistance is associated with hepatocellular carcinoma in chronic hepatitis C infection. World J Gastroenterol. 2010;16:2265–71.
136. Kuriyama S, Miwa Y, Fukushima H, Nakamura H, Toda K, Shiraki M, et al. Prevalence of diabetes and incidence of angiopathy in patients with chronic viral liver disease. J Clin Biochem Nutr. 2007;40:116–22.
137. Fujiwara F, Ishii M, Taneichi H, Miura M, Toshihiro M, Takebe N, et al. Low incidence of vascular complications in patients with diabetes mellitus associated with liver cirrhosis as compared with type 2 diabetes mellitus. Tohoku J Exp Med. 2005;205:327–34.
138. Miyajima I, Kawaguchi T, Fukami A, Nagao Y, Adachi H, Sasaki S, et al. Chronic HCV infection was associated with severe insulin resistance and mild atherosclerosis: a population-based study in an HCV hyperendemic area. J Gastroenterol. 2013;48:93–100.
139. Zuwala-Jagiello J, Pazgan-Simon M, Murawska-Cialowicz E, Simon K. Influence of diabetes on circulating apoptotic microparticles in patients with chronic hepatitis C. In Vivo. 2017;31:1027–34.
140. Leone S, Prosperi M, Costarelli S, Nasta P, Maggiolo F, Di Giambenedetto S, et al. Incidence and predictors of cardiovascular disease, chronic kidney disease, and diabetes in HIV/HCV-coinfected patients who achieved sustained virological response. Eur J Clin Microbiol Infect Dis. 2016;35:1511–20.
141. Zhou YY, Zhou XD, Wu SJ, Hu XQ, Tang B, Poucke SV, et al. Synergistic increase in cardiovascular risk in diabetes mellitus with nonalcoholic fatty liver disease: a meta-analysis. Eur J Gastroenterol Hepatol. 2018;30(6):631–6.
142. Liccardo D, Mosca A, Petroni S, Valente P, Giordano U, Mico AG, et al. The association between retinal microvascular changes, metabolic risk factors, and liver histology in pediatric patients with non-alcoholic fatty liver disease (NAFLD). J Gastroenterol. 2015;50:903–12.
143. Targher G, Lonardo A, Byrne CD. Nonalcoholic fatty liver disease and chronic vascular complications of diabetes mellitus. Nat Rev Endocrinol. 2018;14:99–114.
144. Mantovani A, Zaza G, Byrne CD, Lonardo A, Zoppini G, Bonora E, et al. Nonalcoholic fatty liver disease increases risk of incident chronic kidney disease: a systematic review and meta-analysis. Metabolism. 2018;79:64–76.

145. Guo K, Zhang L, Lu J, Yu H, Wu M, Bao Y, et al. Non-alcoholic fatty liver disease is associated with late but not early atherosclerotic lesions in Chinese inpatients with type 2 diabetes. J Diabetes Complications. 2017;31:80–5.
146. Dallio M, Masarone M, Caprio GG, Di Sarno R, Tuccillo C, Sasso FC, et al. Endocan serum levels in patients with non-alcoholic fatty liver disease with or without type 2 diabetes mellitus: a pilot study. J Gastrointestin Liver Dis. 2017;26:261–8.
147. Goh GB, Pan A, Chow WC, Yuan JM, Koh WP. Association between diabetes mellitus and cirrhosis mortality: the Singapore Chinese Health Study. Liver Int. 2017;37:251–8.
148. Wang YG, Wang P, Wang B, Fu ZJ, Zhao WJ, Yan SL. Diabetes mellitus and poorer prognosis in hepatocellular carcinoma: a systematic review and meta-analysis. PLoS One. 2014;9:e95485.
149. Dyson J, Jaques B, Chattopadyhay D, Lochan R, Graham J, Das D, et al. Hepatocellular cancer: the impact of obesity, type 2 diabetes and a multidisciplinary team. J Hepatol. 2014;60:110–7.
150. Michelotti GA, Machado MV, Diehl AM. NAFLD, NASH and liver cancer. Nat Rev Gastroenterol Hepatol. 2013;10:656–65.
151. Huang TS, Lin CL, Lu MJ, Yeh CT, Liang KH, Sun CC, et al. Diabetes, hepatocellular carcinoma, and mortality in hepatitis C-infected patients: a population-based cohort study. J Gastroenterol Hepatol. 2017;32:1355–62.
152. Younossi ZM, Stepanova M, Saab S, Kalwaney S, Clement S, Henry L, et al. The impact of type 2 diabetes and obesity on the long-term outcomes of more than 85 000 liver transplant recipients in the US. Aliment Pharmacol Ther. 2014;40:686–94.
153. Suzuki K, Endo R, Kohgo Y, Ohtake T, Ueno Y, Kato A, et al. Guidelines on nutritional management in Japanese patients with liver cirrhosis from the perspective of preventing hepatocellular carcinoma. Hepatol Res. 2012;42:621–6.
154. Hashida R, Kawaguchi T, Bekki M, Omoto M, Matsuse H, Nago T, et al. Aerobic vs. resistance exercise in non-alcoholic fatty liver disease: a systematic review. J Hepatol. 2017;66:142–52.
155. Kawaguchi T, Yamagishi S, Sata M. Branched-chain amino acids and pigment epithelium-derived factor: novel therapeutic agents for hepatitis c virus-associated insulin resistance. Curr Med Chem. 2009;16:4843–57.
156. Sakata M, Kawahara A, Kawaguchi T, Akiba J, Taira T, Taniguchi E, et al. Decreased expression of insulin and increased expression of pancreatic transcription factor PDX-1 in islets in patients with liver cirrhosis: a comparative investigation using human autopsy specimens. J Gastroenterol. 2013;48:277–85.
157. Kawaguchi T, Taniguchi E, Morita Y, Shirachi M, Tateishi I, Nagata E, et al. Association of exogenous insulin or sulphonylurea treatment with an increased incidence of hepatoma in patients with hepatitis C virus infection. Liver Int. 2010;30:479–86.
158. Kawaguchi T, Kohjima M, Ichikawa T, Seike M, Ide Y, Mizuta T, et al. The morbidity and associated risk factors of cancer in chronic liver disease patients with diabetes mellitus: a multicenter field survey. J Gastroenterol. 2015;50:333–41.
159. Singh S, Singh PP, Singh AG, Murad MH, Sanchez W. Anti-diabetic medications and the risk of hepatocellular cancer: a systematic review and meta-analysis. Am J Gastroenterol. 2013;108:881–91.. quiz 892
160. Hassan MM, Curley SA, Li D, Kaseb A, Davila M, Abdalla EK, et al. Association of diabetes duration and diabetes treatment with the risk of hepatocellular carcinoma. Cancer. 2010;116:1938–46.
161. Chan KM, Kuo CF, Hsu JT, Chiou MJ, Wang YC, Wu TH, et al. Metformin confers risk reduction for developing hepatocellular carcinoma recurrence after liver resection. Liver Int. 2017;37:434–41.
162. Huang MY, Chung CH, Chang WK, Lin CS, Chen KW, Hsieh TY, et al. The role of thiazolidinediones in hepatocellular carcinoma risk reduction: a population-based cohort study in Taiwan. Am J Cancer Res. 2017;7:1606–16.
163. Singal AG, El-Serag HB. Hepatocellular carcinoma from epidemiology to prevention: translating knowledge into practice. Clin Gastroenterol Hepatol. 2015;13:2140–51.

164. Seo YS, Kim YJ, Kim MS, Suh KS, Kim SB, Han CJ, et al. Association of metformin use with cancer-specific mortality in hepatocellular carcinoma after curative resection: a nationwide population-based study. Medicine (Baltimore). 2016;95:e3527.
165. Smith BK, Marcinko K, Desjardins EM, Lally JS, Ford RJ, Steinberg GR. Treatment of nonalcoholic fatty liver disease: role of AMPK. Am J Physiol Endocrinol Metab. 2016;311:E730–40.
166. Hsu HT, Chi CW. Emerging role of the peroxisome proliferator-activated receptor-gamma in hepatocellular carcinoma. J Hepatocell Carcinoma. 2014;1:127–35.
167. Casadei Gardini A, Faloppi L, De Matteis S, Foschi FG, Silvestris N, Tovoli F, et al. Metformin and insulin impact on clinical outcome in patients with advanced hepatocellular carcinoma receiving sorafenib: validation study and biological rationale. Eur J Cancer. 2017;86:106–14.
168. Casadei Gardini A, Marisi G, Scarpi E, Scartozzi M, Faloppi L, Silvestris N, et al. Effects of metformin on clinical outcome in diabetic patients with advanced HCC receiving sorafenib. Expert Opin Pharmacother. 2015;16:2719–25.
169. Arase Y, Kawamura Y, Seko Y, Kobayashi M, Suzuki F, Suzuki Y, et al. Efficacy and safety in sitagliptin therapy for diabetes complicated by non-alcoholic fatty liver disease. Hepatol Res. 2013;43:1163–8.
170. Fukuhara T, Hyogo H, Ochi H, Fujino H, Kan H, Naeshiro N, et al. Efficacy and safety of sitagliptin for the treatment of nonalcoholic fatty liver disease with type 2 diabetes mellitus. Hepatogastroenterology. 2014;61:323–8.
171. Asakawa M, Mitsui H, Akihisa M, Sekine T, Niitsu Y, Kobayashi A, et al. Efficacy and safety of sitagliptin for the treatment of diabetes mellitus complicated by chronic liver injury. Springerplus. 2015;4:346.
172. Mashitani T, Noguchi R, Okura Y, Namisaki T, Mitoro A, Ishii H, et al. Efficacy of alogliptin in preventing non-alcoholic fatty liver disease progression in patients with type 2 diabetes. Biomed Rep. 2016;4:183–7.
173. Okura Y, Namisaki T, Moriya K, Kitade M, Takeda K, Kaji K, et al. Combined treatment with dipeptidyl peptidase-4 inhibitor (sitagliptin) and angiotensin-II type 1 receptor blocker (losartan) suppresses progression in a non-diabetic rat model of steatohepatitis. Hepatol Res. 2017;47:1317–28.
174. Itou M, Kawaguchi T, Taniguchi E, Sata M. Dipeptidyl peptidase-4: a key player in chronic liver disease. World J Gastroenterol. 2013;19:2298–306.
175. Jojima T, Tomotsune T, Iijima T, Akimoto K, Suzuki K, Aso Y. Empagliflozin (an SGLT2 inhibitor), alone or in combination with linagliptin (a DPP-4 inhibitor), prevents steatohepatitis in a novel mouse model of non-alcoholic steatohepatitis and diabetes. Diabetol Metab Syndr. 2016;8:45.
176. Klein T, Fujii M, Sandel J, Shibazaki Y, Wakamatsu K, Mark M, et al. Linagliptin alleviates hepatic steatosis and inflammation in a mouse model of non-alcoholic steatohepatitis. Med Mol Morphol. 2014;47:137–49.
177. Jung YA, Choi YK, Jung GS, Seo HY, Kim HS, Jang BK, et al. Sitagliptin attenuates methionine/choline-deficient diet-induced steatohepatitis. Diabetes Res Clin Pract. 2014;105:47–57.
178. Hwang HJ, Jung TW, Kim BH, Hong HC, Seo JA, Kim SG, et al. A dipeptidyl peptidase-IV inhibitor improves hepatic steatosis and insulin resistance by AMPK-dependent and JNK-dependent inhibition of LECT2 expression. Biochem Pharmacol. 2015;98:157–66.
179. Ideta T, Shirakami Y, Miyazaki T, Kochi T, Sakai H, Moriwaki H, et al. The dipeptidyl peptidase-4 inhibitor teneligliptin attenuates hepatic lipogenesis via AMPK activation in non-alcoholic fatty liver disease model mice. Int J Mol Sci. 2015;16:29207–18.
180. Wang H, Liu X, Long M, Huang Y, Zhang L, Zhang R, et al. NRF2 activation by antioxidant antidiabetic agents accelerates tumor metastasis. Sci Transl Med. 2016;8:334–51.
181. Harada M, Yoneda A, Haruyama S, Yabuki K, Honma Y, Hiura M, et al. Bullous pemphigoid associated with the dipeptidyl peptidase-4 inhibitor sitagliptin in a patient with liver cirrhosis complicated with rapidly progressive hepatocellular carcinoma. Intern Med. 2017;56:2471–4.
182. Gomez-Peralta F, Abreu C, Lecube A, Bellido D, Soto A, Morales C, et al. Practical approach to initiating SGLT2 inhibitors in type 2 diabetes. Diabetes Ther. 2017;8:953–62.

183. Vallon V, Thomson SC. Targeting renal glucose reabsorption to treat hyperglycaemia: the pleiotropic effects of SGLT2 inhibition. Diabetologia. 2017;60:215–25.
184. Tanaka A, Node K. Emerging roles of sodium-glucose cotransporter 2 inhibitors in cardiology. J Cardiol. 2017;69:501–7.
185. Hayashizaki-Someya Y, Kurosaki E, Takasu T, Mitori H, Yamazaki S, Koide K, et al. Ipragliflozin, an SGLT2 inhibitor, exhibits a prophylactic effect on hepatic steatosis and fibrosis induced by choline-deficient l-amino acid-defined diet in rats. Eur J Pharmacol. 2015;754:19–24.
186. Nakano S, Katsuno K, Isaji M, Nagasawa T, Buehrer B, Walker S, et al. Remogliflozin etabonate improves fatty liver disease in diet-induced obese male mice. J Clin Exp Hepatol. 2015;5:190–8.
187. Qiang S, Nakatsu Y, Seno Y, Fujishiro M, Sakoda H, Kushiyama A, et al. Treatment with the SGLT2 inhibitor luseogliflozin improves nonalcoholic steatohepatitis in a rodent model with diabetes mellitus. Diabetol Metab Syndr. 2015;7:104.
188. Takeda A, Irahara A, Nakano A, Takata E, Koketsu Y, Kimata K, et al. The improvement of the hepatic histological findings in a patient with non-alcoholic steatohepatitis with type 2 diabetes after the administration of the sodium-glucose cotransporter 2 inhibitor ipragliflozin. Intern Med. 2017;56:2739–44.
189. Tobita H, Sato S, Miyake T, Ishihara S, Kinoshita Y. Effects of dapagliflozin on body composition and liver tests in patients with nonalcoholic steatohepatitis associated with type 2 diabetes mellitus: a prospective, open-label, uncontrolled study. Curr Ther Res Clin Exp. 2017;87:13–9.
190. Ito D, Shimizu S, Inoue K, Saito D, Yanagisawa M, Inukai K, et al. Comparison of ipragliflozin and pioglitazone effects on nonalcoholic fatty liver disease in patients with type 2 diabetes: a randomized, 24-week, open-label, active-controlled trial. Diabetes Care. 2017;40:1364–72.
191. Shibuya T, Fushimi N, Kawai M, Yoshida Y, Hachiya H, Ito S, et al. Luseogliflozin improves liver fat deposition compared to metformin in type 2 diabetes patients with non-alcoholic fatty liver disease: a prospective randomized controlled pilot study. Diabetes Obes Metab. 2018;20:438–42.
192. Komiya C, Tsuchiya K, Shiba K, Miyachi Y, Furuke S, Shimazu N, et al. Ipragliflozin improves hepatic steatosis in obese mice and liver dysfunction in type 2 diabetic patients irrespective of body weight reduction. PLoS One. 2016;11:e0151511.
193. Honda Y, Imajo K, Kato T, Kessoku T, Ogawa Y, Tomeno W, et al. The selective SGLT2 inhibitor ipragliflozin has a therapeutic effect on nonalcoholic steatohepatitis in mice. PLoS One. 2016;11:e0146337.
194. Sumida Y, Yoneda M. Current and future pharmacological therapies for NAFLD/NASH. J Gastroenterol. 2018;53(3):362–76.
195. Scafoglio C, Hirayama BA, Kepe V, Liu J, Ghezzi C, Satyamurthy N, et al. Functional expression of sodium-glucose transporters in cancer. Proc Natl Acad Sci U S A. 2015;112:E4111–9.
196. Saito T, Okada S, Yamada E, Shimoda Y, Osaki A, Tagaya Y, et al. Effect of dapagliflozin on colon cancer cell [Rapid Communication]. Endocr J. 2015;62:1133–7.
197. Okada J, Matsumoto S, Kaira K, Saito T, Yamada E, Yokoo H, et al. Sodium glucose cotransporter 2 inhibition combined with cetuximab significantly reduced tumor size and carcinoembryonic antigen level in colon cancer metastatic to liver. Clin Colorectal Cancer. 2018;17(1):e45–8.
198. Obara K, Shirakami Y, Maruta A, Ideta T, Miyazaki T, Kochi T, et al. Preventive effects of the sodium glucose cotransporter 2 inhibitor tofogliflozin on diethylnitrosamine-induced liver tumorigenesis in obese and diabetic mice. Oncotarget. 2017;8:58353–63.
199. Kaji K, Nishimura N, Seki K, Sato S, Saikawa S, Nakanishi K, et al. Sodium glucose cotransporter 2 inhibitor canagliflozin attenuates liver cancer cell growth and angiogenic activity by inhibiting glucose uptake. Int J Cancer. 2017;142(8):1712–22.
200. Tang H, Dai Q, Shi W, Zhai S, Song Y, Han J. SGLT2 inhibitors and risk of cancer in type 2 diabetes: a systematic review and meta-analysis of randomised controlled trials. Diabetologia. 2017;60:1862–72.

201. Donadon V, Balbi M, Casarin P, Vario A, Alberti A. Association between hepatocellular carcinoma and type 2 diabetes mellitus in Italy: potential role of insulin. World J Gastroenterol. 2008;14:5695–700.
202. Donadon V, Balbi M, Ghersetti M, Grazioli S, Perciaccante A, Della Valentina G, et al. Antidiabetic therapy and increased risk of hepatocellular carcinoma in chronic liver disease. World J Gastroenterol. 2009;15:2506–11.
203. Bosetti C, Franchi M, Nicotra F, Asciutto R, Merlino L, La Vecchia C, et al. Insulin and other antidiabetic drugs and hepatocellular carcinoma risk: a nested case-control study based on Italian healthcare utilization databases. Pharmacoepidemiol Drug Saf. 2015;24:771–8.
204. Lee MS, Hsu CC, Wahlqvist ML, Tsai HN, Chang YH, Huang YC. Type 2 diabetes increases and metformin reduces total, colorectal, liver and pancreatic cancer incidences in Taiwanese: a representative population prospective cohort study of 800,000 individuals. BMC Cancer. 2011;11:20.
205. Zhang H, Gao C, Fang L, Zhao HC, Yao SK. Metformin and reduced risk of hepatocellular carcinoma in diabetic patients: a meta-analysis. Scand J Gastroenterol. 2013;48:78–87.
206. Zhang ZJ, Zheng ZJ, Shi R, Su Q, Jiang Q, Kip KE. Metformin for liver cancer prevention in patients with type 2 diabetes: a systematic review and meta-analysis. J Clin Endocrinol Metab. 2012;97:2347–53.
207. Chen TM, Lin CC, Huang PT, Wen CF. Metformin associated with lower mortality in diabetic patients with early stage hepatocellular carcinoma after radiofrequency ablation. J Gastroenterol Hepatol. 2011;26:858–65.

Chapter 8
Obesity and Hepatocarcinogenesis

Yoshio Sumida, Yuya Seko, Tasuku Hara, Akihiko Ohashi, Yukiomi Nakade, Kiyoaki Ito, Haruhisa Nakao, Yoshitaka Fukuzawa, Yoshito Itoh, Takeshi Okanoue, and Masashi Yoneda

Abstract Obesity has been recognized as a cluster of risk factors associated with type 2 diabetes (T2D), cardiovascular morbidity, and higher frequency of cancers in a variety of tissues including the liver. Liver cancer most often occurs as hepatocellular carcinoma (HCC) complicating cirrhosis due to chronic viral infection, heavy alcohol consumption, or non-alcoholic steatohepatitis (NASH) which is a severe form of non-alcoholic fatty liver disease (NAFLD). NAFLD is a major cause of liver disease worldwide, and is becoming the leading cause of HCC/liver transplantation. Obesity-associated HCC has recently been attributed to molecular mechanisms such as chronic inflammation due to adipose tissue remodeling and pro-inflammatory adipokine secretion, ectopic lipid accumulation and lipotoxicity, altered gut microbiota, and disrupted senescence in stellate cells, as well as insulin resistance leading to increased levels of insulin and insulin-like growth factors. Genetic polymorphism has also an important role in the development of HCC without hepatitis virus infection. PNPLA3 genotype GG is the most significant predictor for incident HCC in patients with obesity, T2D, and NAFLD. The frequency of PNPLA3 G allele is known to be more prevalent in Asians and Hispanics than other ethnics. These mechanisms synergize and accelerate the development of HCC before or after the onset of cirrhosis. Better understanding of this complex process will improve our strategies of HCC prevention, prediction, and surveillance in obesity-associated diseases.

Keywords NAFLD · Hepatic fibrosis · PNPLA3 · Type 2 diabetes

Y. Sumida (✉) · A. Ohashi · Y. Nakade · K. Ito · H. Nakao · Y. Fukuzawa · M. Yoneda
Division of Hepatology and Pancreatology, Department of Internal Medicine, Aichi Medical University, Nagakute, Aichi, Japan
e-mail: sumida.yoshio.500@mail.aichi-med-u.ac.jp

Y. Seko · T. Hara · Y. Itoh
Department of Gastroenterology and Hepatology, Kyoto Prefectural University of Medicine, Kyoto, Japan

T. Okanoue
Hepatology Center, Saiseikai Suita Hospital, Suita, Japan

H. Yoshiji, K. Kaji (eds.), *Alcoholic/Non-Alcoholic Digestive Diseases*,
https://doi.org/10.1007/978-981-13-1465-0_8

8.1 Introduction

Hepatocellular carcinoma (HCC) is the fifth most common cancer and the second leading cause of cancer-related death worldwide. The main etiology of HCC has been hepatitis virus infection for several decades. The development of anti-hepatitis viral agents, including direct acting antivirals for hepatitis C virus (HCV) or nucleoside analogues for hepatitis B virus (HBV), can lead to decrease in incidence of HCC worldwide [1]. In Japan, the prevalence of the so-called non-B, non-C HCC (NBNC-HCC) has been increasing. The main causes of NBNC-HCC are lifestyle related diseases such as heavy alcohol consumption or metabolic syndrome [2]. Therefore, Professor Koike at Tokyo University Hospital, the president of the Japan Society of Hepatology (JSH), has suggested that NBNC-HCC mostly consists of the so-called metabolism-associated liver cancer (MALC).We also believe that the main causes of HCC are ABCD (alcohol, HBV, HCV, and diabetes) (Fig. 8.1).

8.1.1 Obesity and HCC

Obesity has become more prevalent in most developed countries over the past few decades [3], and is increasingly recognized as a major risk factor for several common types of cancer, including HCC [4]. In the United States (US), the relative risk of death from HCC in obese patients with body mass index (BMI) $\geq$ 35 kg/m^2 was 4.52 and 1.68 times higher among men and women, respectively, compared with their reference groups [5]. In 5.24 million individuals registered in the Clinical Practice Research Datalink, BMI was significantly associated with liver cancer risk (hazard ratio [HR]: 1.19 per BMI 5 kg/m^2) [4]. According to recent longitudinal data from the Swedish men cohort, overweight in late adolescence was a significant predictor of severe liver disease, including HCC [6, 7]. This risk was enhanced in individuals who develop incident type 2 diabetes (T2D) during the observation period [7]. In Japanese cirrhotic patients, obesity (BMI $\geq$ 25 kg/m^2) was proved to be an independent risk factor for HCC development [8]. Genetic polymorphisms (I148M) in the gene encoding patatin-like phospholipase domain-containing protein 3 (PNPLA3) which is a known risk factor for histologic steatosis as well as non-alcoholic steatohepatitis (NASH), fibrosis, and cirrhosis [9–11] have an increased risk (HR: 5.9; 95% confidence interval (CI) 1.5–23.8; *P*-value = 0.013) of developing HCC in severely obese individuals [12]. Several plausible mechanisms underlying mechanisms of obesity-related hepatocarcinogenesis have been suggested, including

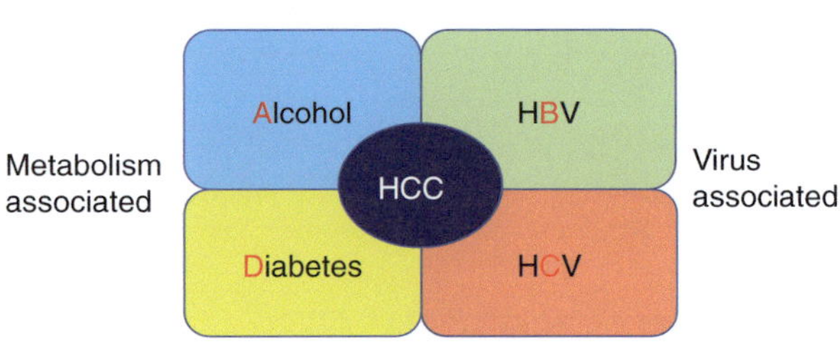

Fig. 8.1 The main causes of HCC are ABCD (alcohol, HBV, HCV, and diabetes)

dysregulated cytokines and adipokines, oxidative stress and endoplasmic reticulum (ER) stress, aberrations in insulin-like growth factor-1 (IGF-1) signaling, and changes in intestinal microbiota (dysbiosis) [13–17].

8.1.2 Diabetes and HCC

An estimated 400 million individuals have diabetes worldwide, among whom 85–95% have T2D. There is emerging evidence of a link between T2D and an increased risk of developing cancer and death from cancer. In a meta-analysis of 13 case–control and 13 cohort studies, diabetes was associated with increased HCC risk (odds ratio[OR]: 2.5 and HR:2.5) [18]. A more recent meta-analysis of 23 cohort studies reported a pooled relative risk (RR) of 2.0 [19]. In recent two large cohorts of US men and women, with over 26 years of follow-up, T2D is significantly associated with incident HCC. This risk was enhanced in patients with a prolonged duration of T2D, and in those with an increasing number of comorbid metabolic conditions (dyslipidemia, obesity [BMI more than 30 kg/m^2], and hypertension) [20]. T2DM was associated with a 26% increased risk of death from any cancer also in Asians. The HR of HCC is 2.05 [21]. In Japan, Nakamura and colleagues demonstrated that HCC was the fifth leading causes of mortality (6.0%) in 45,708 Japanese diabetic patients at 241 hospitals during 2001–2010 [22] (Fig. 8.2).

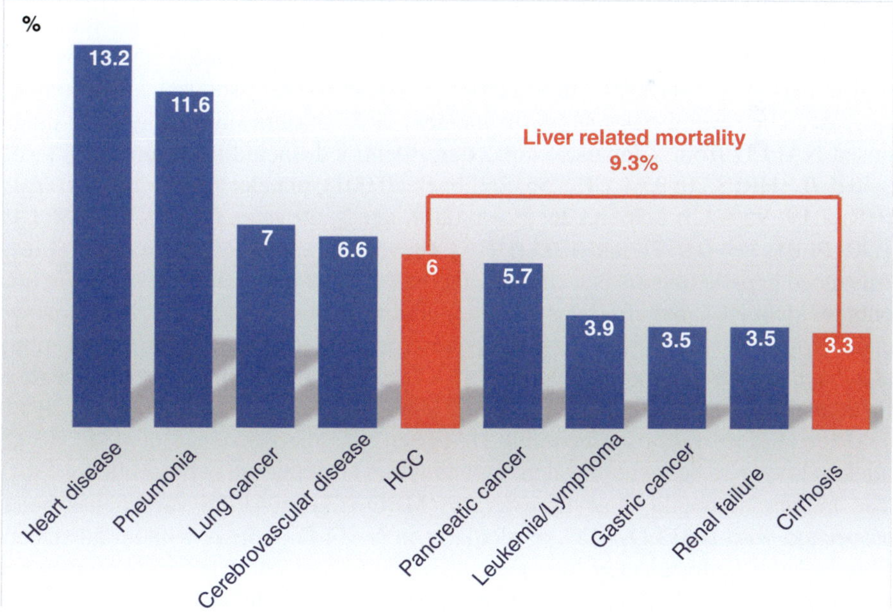

Fig. 8.2 Causes of death in Japanese diabetic patients during 2001–2010 ($n = 45,708$). This figure was originally made in reference to the following paper: Nakamura J, et al. J Diabetes Investig. (2017). Liver-related mortality was the third leading cause (9.3%) of mortality in diabetic patients in Japan

Since the tenth cause is liver cirrhosis (3.3%), 9.3% of diabetic patients totally died from liver-related diseases in Japan.

It is important to identify those patients with T2D who have a high risk of developing HCC. Risk factors for incident HCC in T2D patients have not been established. Three parameters which are associated with HCC incidence are old age (>65 year), low triglyceride level (<150 mg/dL), and high gamma-glutamyl transferase level (>40 IU/L) [23]. A multicenter study from Japan by Korenaga and colleagues demonstrated that the SNPs of PNPLA3 and juxtaposed with another zinc finger protein 1 (JAZF1) were associated with development of HCC in T2DM patients without hepatitis virus infection [24]. That study included 389 T2D patients, including 59 patients with HCC (T2D-HCC) and 330 patients without HCC (T2D-non-HCC). Compared to T2D-non-HCC patients, T2D-HCC patients had the significantly higher frequency of the PNPLA3 G allele (OR = 2.53, $P = 1.05 \times 10^{-5}$). Moreover, among the 115 T2D patients with PNPLA3 genotype GG, HCC patients had a significantly higher frequency of the JAZF1 rs864745 G allele (OR = 3.44, $P = 0.0002$). We conclude that SNPs of PNPLA3 and JAZF1 may be associated with an increased risk of developing HCC among T2D patients without viral hepatitis.

8.1.3 NAFLD and HCC

Non-alcoholic fatty liver disease (NAFLD) is becoming a major cause of HCC, with a steadily rising trend compared to virus-induced chronic hepatitis. One fourth of the adult population is globally affected by NAFLD [25]. In the USA, across the 6-year period (2004–2009), the number of NAFLD-HCC showed a 9% annual increase. The several risk factors for incident HCC in ultrasonography (US) diagnosed NAFLD from a Japanese cohort are identified, including serum AST level ≥40 IU/L (HR: 8.20; 95% CI: 2.56–26.26; $P < 0.001$), platelet count $<150 \times 10^3/\mu L$ (HR: 7.19; 95% CI: 2.26–23.26; $P = 0.001$), age ≥ 60 years (HR: 4.27; 95% CI: 1.30–14.01; $P = 0.017$), and T2D (HR: 3.21; 95% CI: 1.09–9.50; $P = 0.035$) [26]. Advanced hepatic fibrosis is well known to be the most important risk factor for not only incident HCC but also liver-related mortality in NAFLD [27, 28]. T2D is associated with liver fibrosis severity in Japanese patients with NASH [29]. It has now also been shown to be an independent risk factor for development of HCC with a meta-analysis showing that PNPLA3 rs738409 SNP is associated with an OR of 1.40 for HCC in cirrhosis including NAFLD [20]. The frequency of PNPLA3 G allele is known to be more prevalent in Asians and Hispanics than other ethnics [30]. The membrane-bound O-acyltransferase (MBOAT7) rs641738 variant has been associated with NAFLD-HCC, particularly in NAFLD patients without advanced fibrosis [31]. Unfortunately, this phenomenon was not validated in our Japanese multicenter study. We found that dysferlin (DYSF) SNPs located on chromosome 2 in addition to PNPLA3 SNP were also associated with NASH-associated HCC [32]. A recent genome-wide association study found that DYSF SNP was also associated with survival of pancreatic cancer patients [33].

The precise mechanisms underlying carcinogenesis in NAFLD patients remain unknown. Lipotoxicity [34], metabolic or stress response pathways [35], bacterial metabolite (deoxycholic acid)-induced senescence-associated secretory phenotype (SASP)-mediated HSC activation that promotes tumors [14], disruption of circadian rhythm [36], depletion of antitumor CD4+ T-cells by linoleic acid from hepatocytes [37], induction of metabolic inflammation-associated interleukin 17A [38], and prostaglandin E2-mediated suppression of antitumor immunity by gut microbiota [39] are all potential mechanisms of NAFLD carcinogenesis.

On the other hand, the leading mortality of NAFLD patients is cardiovascular diseases (CVD). The second leading cause of NAFLD mortality is extrahepatic neoplasms [40]. In our hospital based cohort of biopsy-proven NAFLD, however, the mortality rate of CVD is very rare but the extrahepatic malignancy is the leading cause of death [27]. In fact, NAFLD showed a strong association with three cancers: HCC (HR 16.73; 95% CI 2.09–133.85; $p = 0.008$), colorectal cancer in males (HR 2.01; 95% CI 1.10–3.68; $p = 0.02$), and breast cancer in females (HR 1.92; 95% CI 1.15–3.20; $p = 0.01$) [41]. A high NAFLD fibrosis score (NFS) and a high fibrosis-4 (FIB-4) score were associated with the development of all cancers and HCC. These three cancers should be screened in NAFLD patients with severe fibrosis.

8.1.4 HCC Surveillance

Poor surveillance is a constant problem for patients with NAFLD. Less patients who were diagnosed with NALD-HCC have received regular surveillance compared to those with HCV-associated HCC [42, 43]. However, the current HCC incidence rate among NAFLD patients was 0.44 (range, 0.29–0.66) per 1000 person-years, and that in NASH was 5.29 (range, 0.75–37.56) per 1000 person-years [25]. The surveillance of every patient with NAFLD is impractical on the view of health economics. HCC surveillance is now recommended only in cirrhotic NAFLD patients by the American Association for the Liver Diseases (AASLD) practice guidance published in 2018 [44], because it is estimated that the risk for HCC in non-cirrhotic NAFLD patients is very small given the large number of NAFLD patients without cirrhosis in the general population. However, the absence of established cirrhosis is more frequently associated with HCC in NAFLD compared to other etiologies, especially in men with NAFLD [45]. In our cohort from data on Japanese patients with biopsy-proven NAFLD, two parameters such as severe hepatic fibrosis (stage 3/4) and PNPLA3 GG genotype were selected as independent predictors for the development of HCC [46] (Fig. 8.3). Therefore we newly suggest that NAFLD patients with fibrosis stage 3/4 or PNPLA3 GG genotype should be screened for HCC. The determination of PNPLA3 genotype might provide patient-risk stratification for tailored HCC surveillance in NAFLD (Fig. 8.4), but it is not considered cost-effective yet. Thus, the EASL-EASD-EASO clinical practice guidelines conclude that extending systematic surveillance to NAFLD patients without cirrhosis

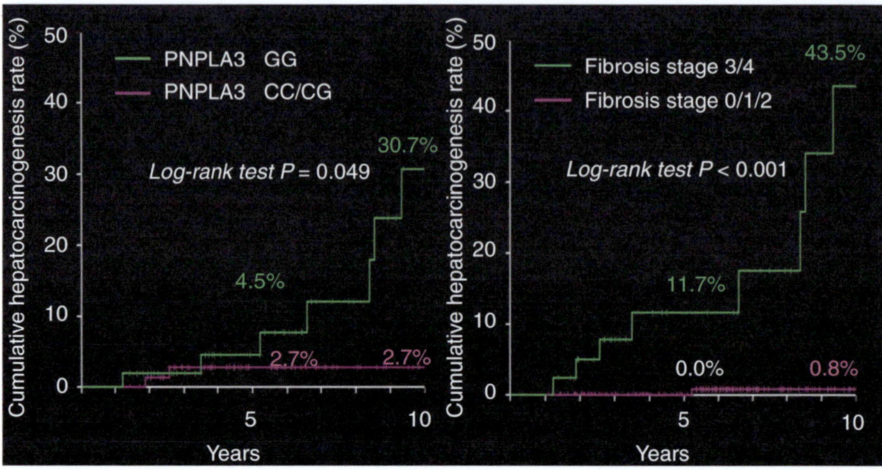

Fig. 8.3 Independent risk factors for incident HCC in Japanese patients with biopsy-proven NAFLD ($n = 238$). PNPLA3 genotype GG and severe hepatic fibrosis (stage 3/4) were selected as independent variables for incident HCC in NAFLD patients by multivariate analysis. This figure was cited from the reference: Seko Y, Sumida Y, et al. Hepatol Res (2017)

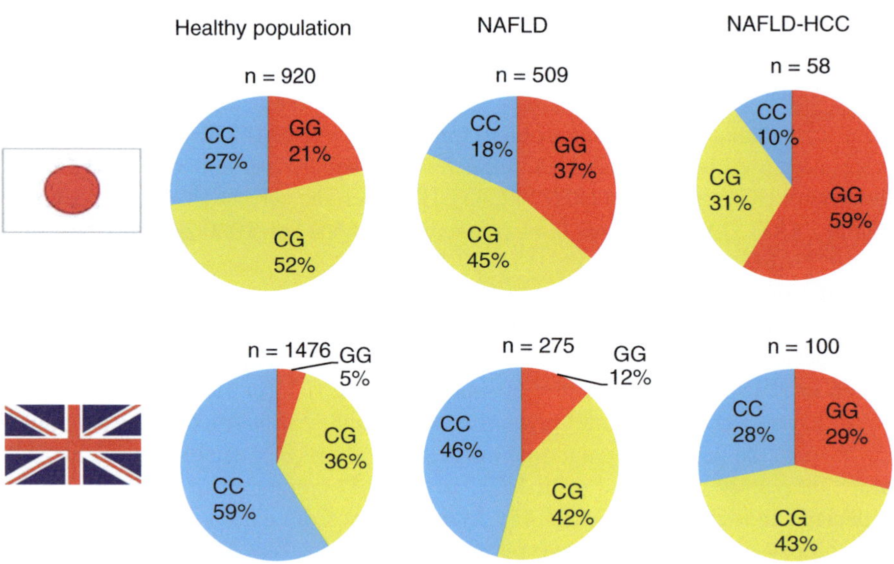

Fig. 8.4 Distribution of PNPLA3 genotype of general population and NAFLD patients with HCC and without in Japan and UK. This figure was originally made in reference to the following papers: Nishioji K, Sumida Y, et al. PLOS One (2016), Seko Y, Sumida Y, et al. Hepatol Res (2017), Liu H, et al. J Hepatol (2014), and Kawaguchi T, Sumida Y, Okanoue T, et al. PLOS One (2018)

would have major cost implications and would need careful consideration [47]. The development of risk scores to guide future surveillance strategies is needed [48].

The next problem is the best modality for HCC surveillance in NAFLD patients. Abdominal US and α-fetoprotein (AFP) have been widely used as the main HCC screening modalities. However, these have several drawbacks for detecting HCC in NAFLD patients. First, US has significant limitations in detection of liver lesions in the presence of obesity and steatosis. The AFP levels are often normal in patients with NASH-HCC. Another tumor marker, des-gamma-carboxy prothrombin (DCP), is elevated in about 60% of NASH-HCC patients [45, 46], although underlying mechanism remains unknown. Recently, integrative scores combining serum biomarkers with clinical variables have been proposed to improve diagnostic performance. GALAD score is now the most valuable scoring systems for predicting incident HCC. The GALAD score was calculated using the published formula: $-10.08 + 0.09 \times \text{age} + 1.67 \times \text{male gender} + 2.34 \times \log(\text{AFP}) + 0.04 \times \text{AFP-L3} + 1.33 \times \log(\text{DCP})$ [49, 50]. The scoring systems should be evaluated for predicting HCC incidence in NAFLD patients.

In Japan, Kawanaka et al. have found that *Wisteria floribunda* agglutinin-positive Mac-2 binding protein, a novel hepatic fibrosis marker [51, 52], is predictor for incident HCC in NAFLD patients [53]. According to another Japanese study by Hiraoka et al., HCC surveillance with US is recommended for T2D patients, especially those who are elderly (≥65 years) and have a high FIB-4 index [54].

Magnetic resonance elastography (MRE) is now known to be the best tool for evaluating hepatic fibrosis among several modalities, including Fibroscan [55]. Although MRE is also useful for predicting development of HCC in patients with chronic liver diseases [56], its usefulness has never been established in NAFLD patients. MRE has several advantages such as accuracy and reproducibility for detecting fibrosis and steatosis, non-invasiveness, measurement of iron content in the liver, and ability of early HCC detection. However, several drawbacks also exist, such as high cost, contraindications for patients with cardiac pacemaker, and a small number of available institutions in Japan.

8.1.5 HCC Prevention

8.1.5.1 Lifestyle Intervention

Lifestyle intervention may serve as first prevention as suggested by observational studies. A meta-analysis of 19 studies, involving 1,290,045 individuals, reported that increased intake of vegetables, but not fruits, may reduce HCC risk (RR, 0.72) [57].

In large-scale cohort or population-based studies, intake of unsaturated fat (HR, 0.71), *n*-3 polyunsaturated fatty acids (PUFAs) (HR, 0.64), eicosapentaenoic acid (EPA) (HR, 0.56), docosapentaenoic acid (DPA) (HR, 0.64), and docosahexaenoic acid (DHA) (HR, 0.56) is associated with lower HCC risk [58, 59]. A recent meta-analysis showed that an extra two cups per day of coffee was associated with a 35%

reduction in the risk of HCC [60]. Exercise is recommended in NAFLD/NASH patients in the guidelines of Europe, AASLD, and Japan [44, 47, 61]. A recent systematic review concludes that not only aerobic exercise but also resistance exercise reduces hepatic steatosis in NAFLD patients [62]. Animal models showed that exercise might reduce HCC incidence without reducing hepatic steatosis [63], although its effect in human NASH should be explored.

8.1.5.2 Medical Interventions

Several commonly prescribed medications seem promising as chemopreventive agents against HCC, including antidiabetic medications, statin, antioxidative agents, aspirin, statin, branched chain amino acid (BCAA), and novel drug pipelines for NASH.

Antidiabetic Medications In a recent meta-analysis, metformin was associated with a 50% reduction in HCC risk, whereas insulin was associated with a 161% increase in risk [64]. This was confirmed in a comparative network meta-analysis of antidiabetic treatments, in which metformin was superior to insulin for HCC risk reduction (RR 0.30, 95% CI 0.18–0.50) [65]. However, its effects for NAFLD/NASH patients are conflicting. On the basis of accumulating evidences, guidelines from USA, Europe, and Japan suggest that pioglitazone (PIO), an insulin sensitizing drug, is now the first-line therapy for T2D patients with NASH [44, 47, 61]. In contrast, the Asia-Pacific Working Party on NAFLD guidelines 2017 do not recommend long-term use of PIO in NASH patients, because of adverse effects (weight gain/edema) or other safety concerns such as increase in myocardial infarction, congestive heart failure, bladder cancer, and bone fracture [66]. Sodium glucose cotransporter 2 (SGLT2) inhibitor, a novel antidiabetic drug, will become the first candidate for the treatment of T2D patients with NAFLD [67], because this agent has a variety of functions, including weight/body fat reduction, significant decrease in ALT levels, prevention of cardiac failure, and renoprotective effects (EMPA-REG outcome, CVR REAL study, and CANVAS program). A few Japanese studies suggest that SGLT2 inhibitors have also antitumor or anticarcinogenic effects in mice NASH models [68–70]. In human studies, recent meta-analysis shows that canagliflozin, an SGLT2 inhibitor, may reduce gastrointestinal cancer incidence [71]. The effect of SGLT2 inhibitor for reducing incidence of HCC in diabetic patients remains unknown. Glucagon-like peptide-1 receptor (GLP-1R) analogues such as liraglutide and dulaglutide have significant efficacies in biochemistry or liver histology for NAFLD/NASH patients in a multicenter, double-blind RCT and two pilot studies [72–74]. Exenatide, a GLP-1RA, has antitumor activities through cAMP-PKA-EGFR-STAT3 axis in obese DEN-treated mice [75]. This result may make GLP-1RA a novel approach to reduce HCC risk in T2D patients, although human studies are now lacking. The clinical study of semaglutide, a novel GLP-1RA, is now ongoing in NASH patients with stage 2/3 fibrosis (NCT02970942) [76].

Statin Increasing data also highlight an important role for statins: in a large meta-analysis of 4298 cases of HCC among 1.5 million patients, the use of statins was associated with a 37% reduction in HCC incidence [77]. This result has also been confirmed in an Asian population [78]. Among a variety of statins, fluvastatin seems to be more effective in reducing HCC risk [79]. All these data suggest that the use of these medications should be encouraged in patients with NAFLD for reasons beyond their metabolic and cardiovascular benefits.

BCAA A multicenter study by the LOTUS group in Japan showed that oral supplementation with BCAAs (leucine, isoleucine, and valine) in 622 cirrhotic patients potentially improves event-free survival and suppresses the incidence of HCC [8, 80]. The risk for HCC was significantly reduced in the BCAA group with obesity and with an AFP level of ≥20 ng/mL [80]. Yoshiji et al. reported that treatment with BCAAs markedly inhibited the cumulative recurrence of HCC in patients with insulin resistance (IR) [homeostasis model assessment (HOMA) -IR >2.5], who received the local curative therapy for HCC [81]. Although it is plausible that BCAA might reduce HCC via ameliorating IR, the efficacy of BCAA in NASH patients is still unknown. In atherogenic and high-fat (Ath + HF) diet-induced NASH model mice, BCAA supplementation significantly improved hepatic steatosis, inflammation, fibrosis, and tumors at 68 weeks [82]. Taken these data into consideration, the chemoprevention effect of BCAA in patients with NASH-cirrhosis is expected.

Pipelines of NASH Advanced Fibrosis Phase 3 study of two drugs in pipeline of NASH is now ongoing for NASH patients with advanced stage fibrosis. Apoptosis signal-regulating kinase 1 (ASK1) is activated by extracellular TNFα, intracellular oxidative or ER stress and initiates the p38/JNK pathway, resulting in apoptosis and fibrosis. Therefore, inhibition of ASK1 has been proposed as a target for the treatment of NASH. An open-label phase 2 trial evaluating the investigational ASK1 inhibitor selonsertib (SEL, GS-4997) alone or in combination with the monoclonal antibody simtuzumab in NASH patients with fibrosis stages 2/3. Patients receiving SEL demonstrated improvements in several measures of liver disease severity, including fibrosis stage, progression to cirrhosis, liver stiffness, and liver fat content [83]. SEL can also significantly improve patient reported outcomes in NASH patients having poor QOL [84]. Thus, international phase 3 trials evaluating SEL among NASH patients with stage 3 (STELLAR3; NCT03053050) or stage 4 (STELLAR4; NCT03053063) are now ongoing. Since ASK1 pathways seem to be associated with hepatocarcinogenesis [85], it is plausible that SEL may influence on tumor incidence of NASH patients. Would you ask us whether ASK1 inhibitor can reduce progression to HCC in several years?

Cenicriviroc (CVC), a C–C motif chemokine receptor-2/5 (CCR2/5) antagonist, has been developed to primarily target inflammation. This agent has also antifibrotic effects and improves insulin sensitivity. Macrophage recruitment through CCR2 into adipose tissue is believed to play a role in the development of IR and T2D. Since administration of CCR2 antagonist resulted in modest improvement in glycemic parameters compared with placebo, its agent is now under development for diabetic patients. CCR5 antagonist impairs the migration, activation, and proliferation of HSC. According to phase 2b trial (CENTAUR study), significant improvement of fibrosis without worsening NASH after 1 year of CVC treatment was found compared with placebo (20% vs. 10%) [86]. Phase 3 evaluation for the treatment of NASH with stage 2/3 fibrosis is now ongoing and recruiting (AURORA study; NCT03028740). AURORA study will determine long-term clinical outcomes composed of histopathologic progression to cirrhosis, liver-related clinical outcomes, and all-cause mortality. Among these agents under development, several medications may be very promising for HCC prevention in obesity-associated conditions. However, well-designed, prospective, population-based cohort studies might provide the best evidence for chemopreventive efficacy of these agents in obese patients.

8.2 Conclusions

Obesity-associated diseases such as T2D and NASH are associated with increased incidence of HCC (as MALC), although the underlying mechanisms remain unknown. A synergistic effect of NASH, obesity, and T2D may play a role in the development of HCC. Worldwide PNPLA3 GG genotype has been known to be the one of the most significant risk factors for HCC incidence in patients with obesity-associated conditions. Innovative pipeline drugs for NASH are currently in development. It is expected that HCC surveillance algorithm and chemoprevention strategy will be established in the near future in order to reduce MALC-related mortality or morbidity.

References

1. Bertuccio P, Turati F, Carioli G, Rodriguez T, La Vecchia C, Malvezzi M, Negri E. Global trends and predictions in hepatocellular carcinoma mortality. J Hepatol. 2017;67(2):302–9.
2. Tateishi R, Okanoue T, Fujiwara N, Okita K, Kiyosawa K, Omata M, Kumada H, Hayashi N, Koike K. Clinical characteristics, treatment, and prognosis of non-B, non-C hepatocellular carcinoma: a large retrospective multicenter cohort study. J Gastroenterol. 2015;50(3):350–60.
3. GBD 2015 Obesity Collaborators, Afshin A, Forouzanfar MH, Reitsma MB, Sur P, Estep K, Lee A, Marczak L, Mokdad AH, Moradi-Lakeh M, Naghavi M, Salama JS, Vos T, Abate KH, Abbafati C, Ahmed MB, Al-Aly Z, Alkerwi A, Al-Raddadi R, Amare AT, Amberbir A, Amegah AK, Amini E, Amrock SM, Anjana RM, Ärnlöv J, Asayesh H, Banerjee A, Barac A, Baye E, Bennett DA, Beyene AS, Biadgilign S, Biryukov S, Bjertness E, Boneya DJ, Campos-Nonato I, Carrero JJ, Cecilio P, Cercy K, Ciobanu LG, Cornaby L, Damtew SA, Dandona L, Dandona R, Dharmaratne SD, Duncan BB, Eshrati B, Esteghamati A, Feigin VL, Fernandes JC, Fürst T, Gebrehiwot TT, Gold A, Gona PN, Goto A, Habtewold TD, Hadush KT, Hafezi-Nejad N, Hay SI, Horino M, Islami F, Kamal R, Kasaeian A, Katikireddi SV, Kengne AP, Kesavachandran CN, Khader YS, Khang YH, Khubchandani J, Kim D, Kim YJ, Kinfu Y, Kosen S, Ku T, Defo BK, Kumar GA, Larson HJ, Leinsalu M, Liang X, Lim SS, Liu P, Lopez AD, Lozano R, Majeed A, Malekzadeh R, Malta DC, Mazidi M, McAlinden C,

McGarvey ST, Mengistu DT, Mensah GA, Mensink GBM, Mezgebe HB, Mirrakhimov EM, Mueller UO, Noubiap JJ, Obermeyer CM, Ogbo FA, Owolabi MO, Patton GC, Pourmalek F, Qorbani M, Rafay A, Rai RK, Ranabhat CL, Reinig N, Safiri S, Salomon JA, Sanabria JR, Santos IS, Sartorius B, Sawhney M, Schmidhuber J, Schutte AE, Schmidt MI, Sepanlou SG, Shamsizadeh M, Sheikhbahaei S, Shin MJ, Shiri R, Shiue I, Roba HS, DAS S, Silverberg JI, Singh JA, Stranges S, Swaminathan S, Tabarés-Seisdedos R, Tadese F, Tedla BA, Tegegne BS, Terkawi AS, Thakur JS, Tonelli M, Topor-Madry R, Tyrovolas S, Ukwaja KN, Uthman OA, Vaezghasemi M, Vasankari T, Vlassov VV, Vollset SE, Weiderpass E, Werdecker A, Wesana J, Westerman R, Yano Y, Yonemoto N, Yonga G, Zaidi Z, Zenebe ZM, Zipkin B, Murray CJL. Health effects of overweight and obesity in 195 countries over 25 years. N Engl J Med. 2017;377(1):13–27.

4. Bhaskaran K, Douglas I, Forbes H, dos-Santos-Silva I, Leon DA, Smeeth L. Body-mass index and risk of 22 specific cancers: a population-based cohort study of 5·24 million UK adults. Lancet. 2014;384(9945):755–65.
5. Calle EE, Rodriguez C, Walker-Thurmond K, Thun MJ. N Engl J Med. 2003;348:1625–38.
6. Hagström H, Stål P, Hultcrantz R, Hemmingsson T, Andreasson A. Overweight in late adolescence predicts development of severe liver disease later in life: a 39years follow-up study. J Hepatol. 2016;65(2):363–8.
7. Hagström H, Tynelius P, Rasmussen F. High BMI in late adolescence predicts future severe liver disease and hepatocellular carcinoma: a national, population-based cohort study in 1.2 million men. Gut. 2018;67:1536–42. https://doi.org/10.1136/gutjnl-2016-313622.
8. Muto Y, Sato S, Watanabe A, Moriwaki H, Suzuki K, Kato A, Kato M, Nakamura T, Higuchi K, Nishiguchi S, Kumada H, Long-Term Survival Study Group. Effects of oral branched-chain amino acid granules on event-free survival in patients with liver cirrhosis. Clin Gastroenterol Hepatol. 2005;3(7):705–13.
9. Kawaguchi T, Sumida Y, Umemura A, Matsuo K, Takahashi M, Takamura T, Yasui K, Saibara T, Hashimoto E, Kawanaka M, Watanabe S, Kawata S, Imai Y, Kokubo M, Shima T, Park H, Tanaka H, Tajima K, Yamada R, Matsuda F, Okanoue T, Japan Study Group of Nonalcoholic Fatty Liver Disease. Genetic polymorphisms of the human PNPLA3 gene are strongly associated with severity of non-alcoholic fatty liver disease in Japanese. PLoS One. 2012;7(6):e38322.
10. Eslam M, Valenti L, Romeo S. Genetics and epigenetics of NAFLD and NASH: clinical impact. J Hepatol. 2018;68(2):268–79.
11. Singal AG, Manjunath H, Yopp AC, Beg MS, Marrero JA, Gopal P, Waljee AK. The effect of PNPLA3 on fibrosis progression and development of hepatocellular carcinoma: a meta-analysis. Am J Gastroenterol. 2014;109(3):325–34.
12. Burza MA, Pirazzi C, Maglio C, Sjöholm K, Mancina RM, Svensson PA, Jacobson P, Adiels M, Baroni MG, Borén J, Ginanni Corradini S, Montalcini T, Sjöström L, Carlsson LM, Romeo S. PNPLA3 I148M (rs738409) genetic variant is associated with hepatocellular carcinoma in obese individuals. Dig Liver Dis. 2012;44(12):1037–41.
13. Nakagawa H, Umemura A, Taniguchi K, Font-Burgada J, Dhar D, Ogata H, Zhong Z, Valasek MA, Seki E, Hidalgo J, Koike K, Kaufman RJ, Karin M. ER stress cooperates with hypernutrition to trigger TNF-dependent spontaneous HCC development. Cancer Cell. 2014;26(3):331–43.
14. Yoshimoto S, Loo TM, Atarashi K, Kanda H, Sato S, Oyadomari S, Iwakura Y, Oshima K, Morita H, Hattori M, Honda K, Ishikawa Y, Hara E, Ohtani N. Obesity-induced gut microbial metabolite promotes liver cancer through senescence secretome. Nature. 2013;499(7456):97–101. https://doi.org/10.1038/nature12347. Epub 2013 Jun 26
15. Neuschwander-Tetri BA. Non-alcoholic fatty liver disease. BMC Med. 2017;15:45.
16. Park EJ, Lee JH, Yu GY, et al. Dietary and genetic obesity promote liver inflammation and tumorigenesis by enhancing IL-6 and TNF expression. Cell. 2010;140:197–208.
17. Tilg H, Hotamisligil GS. Nonalcoholic fatty liver disease: cytokine-adipokine interplay and regulation of insulin resistance. Gastroenterology. 2006;131:934–45.

18. El-Serag HB, Hampel H, Javadi F. The association between diabetes and hepatocellular carcinoma: a systematic review of epidemiologic evidence. Clin Gastroenterol Hepatol. 2006;4:369–80.
19. Wang C, Wang X, Gong G, et al. Increased risk of hepatocellular carcinoma in patients with diabetes mellitus: a systematic review and meta-analysis of cohort studies. Int J Cancer. 2012;130:1639–48.
20. Simon TG, King LY, Chong DQ, Nguyen L, Ma Y, VoPham T, Giovannucci EL, Fuchs CS, Meyerhardt JA, Corey KE, Khalili H, Chung RT, Zhang X, Chan AT. Diabetes, metabolic comorbidities and risk of hepatocellular carcinoma: results from two prospective cohort studies. Hepatology. 2017;67:1797. https://doi.org/10.1002/hep.29660. [Epub ahead of print].
21. Chen Y, Wu F, Saito E, Lin Y, Song M, Luu HN, Gupta PC, Sawada N, Tamakoshi A, Shu XO, Koh WP, Xiang YB, Tomata Y, Sugiyama K, Park SK, Matsuo K, Nagata C, Sugawara Y, Qiao YL, You SL, Wang R, Shin MH, Pan WH, Pednekar MS, Tsugane S, Cai H, Yuan JM, Gao YT, Tsuji I, Kanemura S, Ito H, Wada K, Ahn YO, Yoo KY, Ahsan H, Chia KS, Boffetta P, Zheng W, Inoue M, Kang D, Potter JD. Association between type 2 diabetes and risk of cancer mortality: a pooled analysis of over 771,000 individuals in the Asia Cohort Consortium. Diabetologia. 2017;60(6):1022–32.
22. Nakamura J, Kamiya H, Haneda M, Inagaki N, Tanizawa Y, Araki E, Ueki K, Nakayama T. Causes of death in Japanese patients with diabetes based on the results of a survey of 45,708 cases during 2001-2010: report of the Committee on Causes of Death in Diabetes Mellitus. J Diabetes Investig. 2017;8(3):397–410.
23. Si WK, Chung JW, Cho J, Baeg JY, Jang ES, Yoon H, Kim J, Shin CM, Park YS, Hwang JH, Jeong SH, Kim N, Lee DH, Lim S, Kim JW. Predictors of Increased Risk of Hepatocellular Carcinoma in Patients with Type 2 Diabetes. PLoS One. 2016;11(6):e0158066.
24. Ueyama M, Nishida N, Korenaga M, Korenaga K, Kumagai E, Yanai H, Adachi H, Katsuyama H, Moriyama S, Hamasaki H, Sako A, Sugiyama M, Aoki Y, Imamura M, Murata K, Masaki N, Kawaguchi T, Torimura T, Hyogo H, Aikata H, Ito K, Sumida Y, Kanazawa A, Watada H, Okamoto K, Honda K, Kon K, Kanto T, Mizokami M, Watanabe S. The impact of PNPLA3 and JAZF1 on hepatocellular carcinoma in non-viral hepatitis patients with type 2 diabetes mellitus. J Gastroenterol. 2016;51(4):370–9.
25. Younossi ZM, Koenig AB, Abdelatif D, et al. Global epidemiology of nonalcoholic fatty liver disease—meta-analytic assessment of prevalence, incidence, and outcomes. Hepatology. 2016;64:73–84.
26. Kawamura Y, Arase Y, Ikeda K, Seko Y, Imai N, Hosaka T, Kobayashi M, Saitoh S, Sezaki H, Akuta N, Suzuki F, Suzuki Y, Ohmoto Y, Amakawa K, Tsuji H, Kumada H. Large-scale long-term follow-up study of Japanese patients with non-alcoholic Fatty liver disease for the onset of hepatocellular carcinoma. Am J Gastroenterol. 2012;107(2):253–61.
27. Seko Y, Sumida Y, Tanaka S, Taketani H, Kanemasa K, Ishiba H, Okajima A, Nishimura T, Yamaguchi K, Moriguchi M, Mitsuyoshi H, Yasui K, Minami M, Itoh Y. Predictors of malignancies and overall mortality in Japanese patients with biopsy-proven non-alcoholic fatty liver disease. Hepatol Res. 2015;45(7):728–38.
28. Dulai PS, Singh S, Patel J, Soni M, Prokop LJ, Younossi Z, Sebastiani G, Ekstedt M, Hagstrom H, Nasr P, Stal P, Wong VW, Kechagias S, Hultcrantz R, Loomba R. Increased risk of mortality by fibrosis stage in nonalcoholic Fatty liver disease: systematic review and meta-analysis. Hepatology. 2017;65(5):1557–65.
29. Nakahara T, Hyogo H, Yoneda M, Sumida Y, Eguchi Y, Fujii H, Ono M, Kawaguchi T, Imajo K, Aikata H, Tanaka S, Kanemasa K, Fujimoto K, Anzai K, Saibara T, Sata M, Nakajima A, Itoh Y, Chayama K, Okanoue T, Japan Study Group of Nonalcoholic Fatty Liver Disease. Type 2 diabetes mellitus is associated with the fibrosis severity in patients with nonalcoholic fatty liver disease in a large retrospective cohort of Japanese patients. J Gastroenterol. 2014;49(11):1477–84.
30. Younossi Z, Anstee QM, Marietti M, Hardy T, Henry L, Eslam M, George J, Bugianesi E. Global burden of NAFLD and NASH: trends, predictions, risk factors and prevention. Nat Rev Gastroenterol Hepatol. 2018;15(1):11–20.

31. Donati B, Dongiovanni P, Romeo S, Meroni M, McCain M, Miele L, et al. MBOAT7 rs641738 variant and hepatocellular carcinoma in noncirrhotic individuals. Sci Rep. 2017;7:4492.
32. Kawaguchi T, Shima T, Mizuno M, Mitsumoto Y, Umemura A, Kanbara Y, Tanaka S, Sumida Y, Yasui K, Takahashi M, Matsuo K, ItohY TK, Hashimoto E, Kiyosawa K, Kawaguchi M, Itoh H, Uto H, Komorizono Y, Shirabe K, Takami S, Takamura T, Kawanaka M, Yamada R, Matsuda F, Okanoue T. Risk estimation model for nonalcoholic fatty liver disease in the Japanese using multiple genetic markers. PLoS One. 2018;13(1):e0185490.
33. Tang H, Wei P, Chang P, Li Y, Yan D, Liu C, Hassan M, Li D. Genetic polymorphisms associated with pancreatic cancer survival: a genome-wide association study. Int J Cancer. 2017;141(4):678–86.
34. Baffy G, Brunt EM, Caldwell SH. Hepatocellular carcinoma in non-alcoholic fatty liver disease: an emerging menace. J Hepatol. 2012;56:1384–91.
35. Michelotti GA, Machado MV, Diehl AM. NAFLD, NASH and liver cancer. Nat Rev Gastroenterol Hepatol. 2013;10:656–65.
36. Kettner NM, Voicu H, Finegold MJ, et al. Circadian homeostasis of liver metabolism suppresses hepatocarcinogenesis. Cancer Cell. 2016;30:909–24.
37. Ma C, Kesarwala AH, Eggert T, et al. NAFLD causes selective CD4(+) T lymphocyte loss and promotes hepatocarcinogenesis. Nature. 2016;531:253–7.
38. Gomes AL, Teijeiro A, Buren S, et al. Metabolic inflammation-associated IL-17A causes nonalcoholic steatohepatitis and hepatocellular carcinoma. Cancer Cell. 2016;30:161–75.
39. Loo TM, Kamachi F, Watanabe Y, et al. Gut microbiota promotes obesity-associated liver cancer through PGE2-mediated suppression of antitumor immunity. Cancer Discov. 2017; 7:522–38.
40. Ong JP, Pitts A, Younossi ZM. Increased overall mortality and liver-related mortality in nonalcoholic fatty liver disease. J Hepatol. 2008;49(4):608–12.
41. Kim GA, Lee HC, Choe J, Kim MJ, Lee MJ, Chang HS, Bae IY, Kim HK, An J, Shim JH, Kim KM, Lim YS. Association between non-alcoholic fatty liver disease and cancer incidence rate. J Hepatol. 2017; https://doi.org/10.1016/j.jhep.2017.09.012.
42. Piscaglia F, Svegliati-Baroni G, Barchetti A. HCC-NAFLD Italian Study Group Clinical patterns of hepatocellular carcinoma in nonalcoholic fatty liver disease: a multicenter prospective study. Hepatology. 2016;63:827–38.
43. Mittal S, Sada Y, El-Serag HB, Kanwal F, Duan Z, Temple S, et al. Temporal trends of nonalcoholic fatty liver disease-related hepatocellular carcinoma in the veteran affairs population. Clin Gastroenterol Hepatol. 2015;13:594–601.
44. Chalasani N, Younossi Z, Lavine JE, Charlton M, Cusi K, Rinella M, Harrison SA, Brunt EM, Sanyal AJ. The diagnosis and management of nonalcoholic fatty liver disease: practice guidance from the American Association for the Study of Liver Diseases. Hepatology. 2018;67(1):328–57. https://doi.org/10.1002/hep.29367. Epub 2017 Sep 29
45. Yasui K, Hashimoto E, Komorizono Y, Koike K, Arii S, Imai Y, Shima T, Kanbara Y, Saibara T, Mori T, Kawata S, Uto H, Takami S, Sumida Y, Takamura T, Kawanaka M, Okanoue T, Japan NASH Study Group, Ministry of Health, Labour, and Welfare of Japan. Characteristics of patients with nonalcoholic steatohepatitis who develop hepatocellular carcinoma. Clin Gastroenterol Hepatol. 2011;9(5):428–33.
46. Seko Y, Sumida Y, Tanaka S, Mori K, Taketani H, Ishiba H, Hara T, Okajima A, Umemura A, Nishikawa T, Yamaguchi K, Moriguchi M, Kanemasa K, Yasui K, Imai S, Shimada K, Itoh Y. Development of hepatocellular carcinoma in Japanese patients with biopsy-proven nonalcoholic fatty liver disease: association between PNPLA3 genotype and hepatocarcinogenesis/fibrosis progression. Hepatol Res. 2017;47(11):1083–92.
47. European Association for the Study of the Liver (EASL), European Association for the Study of Diabetes (EASD), European Association for the Study of Obesity (EASO). EASL-EASD-EASO clinical practice guidelines for the management of non-alcoholic fatty liver disease. J Hepatol. 2016;64:1388–402.
48. Younes R, Bugianesi E. Should we undertake surveillance for HCC in patients with NAFLD? J Hepatol. 2018;68:326–34.

49. Johnson PJ, Pirrie SJ, Cox TF, Berhane S, Teng M, Palmer D, Morse J, Hull D, Patman G, Kagebayashi C, Hussain S, Graham J, Reeves H, Satomura S. The detection of hepatocellular carcinoma using a prospectively developed and validated model based on serological biomarkers. Cancer Epidemiol Biomark Prev. 2014;23(1):144–53.
50. Berhane S, Toyoda H, Tada T, Kumada T, Kagebayashi C, Satomura S, Schweitzer N, Vogel A, Manns MP, Benckert J, Berg T, Ebker M, Best J, Dechêne A, Gerken G, Schlaak JF, Weinmann A, Wörns MA, Galle P, Yeo W, Mo F, Chan SL, Reeves H, Cox T, Johnson P. Role of the GALAD and BALAD-2 serologic models in diagnosis of hepatocellular carcinoma and prediction of survival in patients. Clin Gastroenterol Hepatol. 2016;14(6):875–86.
51. Ito K, Murotani K, Nakade Y, Inoue T, Nakao H, Sumida Y, Kamada Y, Yoneda M. Serum *Wisteria floribunda* agglutinin-positive Mac-2-binding protein levels and liver fibrosis: a meta-analysis. J Gastroenterol Hepatol. 2017;32(12):1922–30.
52. Abe M, Miyake T, Kuno A, Imai Y, Sawai Y, Hino K, Hara Y, Hige S, Sakamoto M, Yamada G, Kage M, Korenaga M, Hiasa Y, Mizokami M, Narimatsu H. Association between *Wisteria floribunda* agglutinin-positive Mac-2 binding protein and the fibrosis stage of non-alcoholic fatty liver disease. J Gastroenterol. 2015;50(7):776–84.
53. Yoneda M, Imajo K, Takahashi H, Ogawa Y, Eguchi Y, Sumida Y, Yoneda M, Kawanaka M, Saito S, Tokushige K, Nakajima A. Clinical strategy of diagnosing and following patients with nonalcoholic fatty liver disease based on invasive and noninvasive methods. J Gastroenterol. 2018;53:181–96. https://doi.org/10.1007/s00535-017-1414-2. [Epub ahead of print]
54. Hiraoka A, Ochi M, Matsuda R, Aibiki T, Okudaira T, Kawamura T, Yamago H, Nakahara H, Suga Y, Azemoto N, Miyata H, Miyamoto Y, Ninomiya T, Hirooka M, Abe M, Matsuura B, Hiasa Y, Michitaka K. Ultrasonography screening for hepatocellular carcinoma in Japanese patients with diabetes mellitus. J Diabetes. 2016;8(5):640–6.
55. Imajo K, Kessoku T, Honda Y, Tomeno W, Ogawa Y, Mawatari H, Fujita K, Yoneda M, Taguri M, Hyogo H, Sumida Y, Ono M, Eguchi Y, Inoue T, Yamanaka T, Wada K, Saito S, Nakajima A. Magnetic resonance imaging more accurately classifies steatosis and fibrosis in patients with nonalcoholic fatty liver disease than transient elastography. Gastroenterology. 2016;150(3):626–37.
56. Motosugi U, Ichikawa T, Koshiishi T, Sano K, Morisaka H, Ichikawa S, Enomoto N, Matsuda M, Fujii H, Araki T. Liver stiffness measured by magnetic resonance elastography as a risk factor for hepatocellular carcinoma: a preliminary case-control study. Eur Radiol. 2013;23(1):156–62.
57. Yang Y, Zhang D, Feng N, et al. Increased intake of vegetables, but not fruit, reduces risk for hepatocellular carcinoma: a meta-analysis. Gastroenterology. 2014;147:1031–42.
58. Duarte-Salles T, Fedirko V, Stepien M, et al. Dietary fat, fat subtypes and hepatocellular carcinoma in a large European cohort. Int J Cancer. 2015;137:2715–28.
59. Sawada N, Inoue M, Iwasaki M, et al. Consumption of n-3 fatty acids and fish reduces risk of hepatocellular carcinoma. Gastroenterology. 2012;142:1468–75.
60. Kennedy OJ, Roderick P, Buchanan R, Fallowfield JA, Hayes PC, Parkes J. Coffee, including caffeinated and decaffeinated coffee, and the risk of hepatocellular carcinoma: a systematic review and dose-response meta-analysis. BMJ Open. 2017;7(5):e013739. https://doi.org/10.1136/bmjopen-2016-013739.
61. Watanabe S, Hashimoto E, Ikejima K, Uto H, Ono M, Sumida Y, Seike M, Takei Y, Takehara T, Tokushige K, Nakajima A, Yoneda M, Saibara T, Shiota G, Sakaida I, Nakamuta M, Mizuta T, Tsubouchi H, Sugano K, Shimosegawa T, Japanese Society of Gastroenterology; Japan Society of Hepatology. Evidence-based clinical practice guidelines for nonalcoholic fatty liver disease/nonalcoholic steatohepatitis. J Gastroenterol. 2015;50(4):364–77.
62. Hashida R, Kawaguchi T, Bekki M, Omoto M, Matsuse H, Nago T, Takano Y, Ueno T, Koga H, George J, Shiba N, Torimura T. Aerobic vs. resistance exercise in non-alcoholic fatty liver disease: a systematic review. J Hepatol. 2017;66(1):142–52.
63. Piguet AC, Saran U, Simillion C, Keller I, Terracciano L, Reeves HL, Dufour JF. Regular exercise decreases liver tumors development in hepatocyte-specific PTEN-deficient mice independently of steatosis. J Hepatol. 2015;62(6):1296–303.

64. Singh S, Singh PP, Singh AG, et al. Anti-diabetic medications and the risk of hepatocellular cancer: a systematic review and meta-analysis. Am J Gastroenterol. 2013;108:881–91.. quiz 892
65. Zhou YY, Zhu GQ, Liu T, et al. Systematic review with network meta-analysis: antidiabetic medication and risk of hepatocellular carcinoma. Sci Rep. 2016;6:33743.
66. Chitturi S, Wong VW, Chan WK, Wong GL, Wong SK, Sollano J, Ni YH, Liu CJ, Lin YC, Lesmana LA, Kim SU, Hashimoto E, Hamaguchi M, Goh KL, Fan J, Duseja A, Dan YY, Chawla Y, Farrell G, Chan HL. The Asia-Pacific working party on non-alcoholic fatty liver disease guidelines 2017-part 2: management and special groups. J Gastroenterol Hepatol. 2018;33(1):86–98.
67. Sumida Y, Seko Y, Yoneda M, Japan Study Group of NAFLD (JSG-NAFLD). Novel antidiabetic medications for non-alcoholic fatty liver disease with type 2 diabetes mellitus. Hepatol Res. 2017;47(4):266–80.
68. Kaji K, Nishimura N, Seki K, Sato S, Saikawa S, Nakanishi K, Furukawa M, Kawaratani H, Kitade M, Moriya K, Namisaki T, Yoshiji H. Sodium glucose cotransporter 2 inhibitor canagliflozin attenuates liver cancer cell growth and angiogenic activity by inhibiting glucose uptake. Int J Cancer. 2018;142:1712. https://doi.org/10.1002/ijc.31193. [Epub ahead of print].
69. Obara K, Shirakami Y, Maruta A, Ideta T, Miyazaki T, Kochi T, Sakai H, Tanaka T, Seishima M, Shimizu M. Preventive effects of the sodium glucose cotransporter 2 inhibitor tofogliflozin on diethylnitrosamine-induced liver tumorigenesis in obese and diabetic mice. Oncotarget. 2017;8(35):58353–63.
70. Shiba K, Tsuchiya K, Komiya C, Miyachi Y, Mori K, Shimazu N, Yamaguchi S, Ogasawara N, Katoh M, Itoh M, Suganami T, Ogawa Y. Canagliflozin, an SGLT2 inhibitor, attenuates the development of hepatocellular carcinoma in a mouse model of human NASH. Sci Rep. 2018;8(1):2362.
71. Tang H, Dai Q, Shi W, Zhai S, Song Y, Han J. SGLT2 inhibitors and risk of cancer in type 2 diabetes: a systematic review and meta-analysis of randomised controlled trials. Diabetologia. 2017;60(10):1862–72.
72. Armstrong MJ, Gaunt P, Aithal GP, Barton D, Hull D, Parker R, Hazlehurst JM, Guo K, LEAN Trial Team, Abouda G, Aldersley MA, Stocken D, Gough SC, Tomlinson JW, Brown RM, Hübscher SG, Newsome PN, Wilku M, Russell C, Iqbal S, Corbett C, Lee MY, Keely J, Nicholls M, Henry S, Lewis M, Dixon E, Myers S, Sharman S, Bishop R. Liraglutide safety and efficacy in patients with non-alcoholic steatohepatitis (LEAN): a multicentre, double-blind, randomised, placebo-controlled phase 2 study. Lancet. 2016;387(10019):679–90.
73. Eguchi Y, Kitajima Y, Hyogo H, Takahashi H, Kojima M, Ono M, Araki N, Tanaka K, Yamaguchi M, Matsuda Y, Ide Y, Otsuka T, Ozaki I, Ono N, Eguchi T, Anzai K, Japan Study Group for NAFLD (JSG-NAFLD). Pilot study of liraglutide effects in non-alcoholic steatohepatitis and non-alcoholic fatty liver disease with glucose intolerance in Japanese patients (LEAN-J). Hepatol Res. 2015;45(3):269–78.
74. Seko Y, Sumida Y, Tanaka S, Mori K, Taketani H, Ishiba H, Hara T, Okajima A, Umemura A, Nishikawa T, Yamaguchi K, Moriguchi M, Kanemasa K, Yasui K, Imai S, Shimada K, Itoh Y. Effect of 12-week dulaglutide therapy in Japanese patients with biopsy-proven non-alcoholic fatty liver disease and type 2 diabetes mellitus. Hepatol Res. 2017;47(11):1206–11.
75. Zhou M, Mok MT, Sun H, Chan AW, Huang Y, Cheng AS, Xu G. The anti-diabetic drug exenatide, a glucagon-like peptide-1 receptor agonist,counteracts hepatocarcinogenesis through cAMP-PKA-EGFR-STAT3 axis. Oncogene. 2017;36(29):4135–49.
76. Katsiki N, Athyros VG, Karagiannis A, Mikhailidis DP. Semaglutide, lipid-lowering drugs, and NAFLD. Lancet Diabetes Endocrinol. 2017;5(5):329–30.
77. Singh S, Singh PP, Singh AG, Murad MH, Sanchez W. Statins are associated with a reduced risk of hepatocellular cancer: a systematic review and meta-analysis. Gastroenterology. 2013;144:323–32.
78. Kim G, Jang SY, Nam CM, Kang ES. Statin use and the risk of hepatocellular carcinoma in patients at high risk: A nationwide nested case-control study. J Hepatol. 2018;53:181–96.

79. Zhou YY, Zhu GQ, Wang Y, Zheng JN, Ruan LY, Cheng Z, Hu B, Fu SW, Zheng MH. Systematic review with network meta-analysis: statins and risk of hepatocellular carcinoma. Oncotarget. 2016;7(16):21753–62. https://doi.org/10.18632/oncotarget.7832.
80. Muto Y, Sato S, Watanabe A, Moriwaki H, Suzuki K, Kato A, Kato M, Nakamura T, Higuchi K, Nishiguchi S, Kumada H, Ohashi Y, Long-Term Survival Study (LOTUS) Group. Overweight and obesity increase the risk for liver cancer in patients with liver cirrhosis and long-term oral supplementation with branched-chain amino acid granules inhibits liver carcinogenesis in heavier patients with liver cirrhosis. Hepatol Res. 2006;35(3):204–14.
81. Yoshiji H, Noguchi R, Namisaki T, Moriya K, Kitade M, Aihara Y, Douhara A, Yamao J, Fujimoto M, Toyohara M, Mitoro A, Sawai M, Yoshida M, Morioka C, Uejima M, Uemura M, Fukui H. Branched-chain amino acids suppress the cumulative recurrence of hepatocellular carcinoma under conditions of insulin-resistance. Oncol Rep. 2013;30(2):545–52.
82. Takegoshi K, Honda M, Okada H, Takabatake R, Matsuzawa-Nagata N, Campbell JS, Nishikawa M, Shimakami T, Shirasaki T, Sakai Y, Yamashita T, Takamura T, Tanaka T, Kaneko S. Branched-chain amino acids prevent hepatic fibrosis and development of hepatocellular carcinoma in a non-alcoholic steatohepatitis mouse model. Oncotarget. 2017;8(11):18191–205.
83. Loomba R, Lawitz E, Mantry PS, et al. The ASK1 inhibitor selonsertib in patients with nonalcoholic steatohepatitis: a randomized, phase 2 trial. Hepatology. In press; https://doi.org/10.1002/hep.29514.
84. Nakagawa H, Hirata Y, Takeda K, Hayakawa Y, Sato T, Kinoshita H, Sakamoto K, Nakata W, Hikiba Y, Omata M, Yoshida H, Koike K, Ichijo H, Maeda S. Apoptosis signal-regulating kinase 1 inhibits hepatocarcinogenesis by controlling the tumor-suppressing function of stress-activated mitogen-activated protein kinase. Hepatology. 2011;54(1):185–95.
85. Younossi ZM, Stepanova M, Lawitz E, Charlton M, Loomba R, Myers RP, Subramanian GM, McHutchison JG, Goodman Z. Improvement of hepatic fibrosis and patient-reported outcomes in non-alcoholic steatohepatitis treated with selonsertib. Liver Int. 2018;38:1849. https://doi.org/10.1111/liv.13706. [Epub ahead of print].
86. Friedman SL, Ratziu V, Harrison SA, et al. A randomized, placebo-controlled trial of cenicriviroc for treatment of nonalcoholic steatohepatitis with fibrosis. Hepatology. In press;

Chapter 9
Microbiota in Non-alcoholic Liver Disease

Yuji Ogawa, Yasushi Honda, Takaomi Kessoku, Wataru Tomeno, Kento Imajo, Masato Yoneda, Satoru Saito, and Atsushi Nakajima

Abstract The liver is exposed to large amounts of bacterial components and metabolites from the intestine. The gut microbiota has recently evolved as an important player in the gut-liver axis. Various liver disorders, including alcoholic liver disease, non-alcoholic fatty liver disease (NAFLD), and primary sclerosing cholangitis, have been reported to be associated with alterations of the gut microbiota. Dysbiosis and a leaky gut are believed to be involved in the pathophysiology of many liver diseases through multiple interactions with the host's immune system and other cell types. Furthermore, it is believed that hyperresponsiveness of the liver to low-dose lipopolysaccharides arriving from the intestine through the portal vein accelerates the pathophysiology of NAFLD. The short-chain fatty acids produced by gut microorganisms are speculated to contribute to liver disease progression via multiple mechanisms. A number of trials focusing on the gut microbiota are currently ongoing. A greater understanding in the future of the involvement of gut microbiota and its components in the pathogenesis of liver diseases might pave the way for the development of novel therapies for these diseases.

Keywords Microbiota · Non-alcoholic fatty liver disease · Primary sclerosing cholangitis

9.1 Introduction

Gut microbiota is defined as the complex mix of microorganisms harbored in the gut of every individual and is characterized by a collection of a large mixture of genes collectively called the microbiome. Normal human gut is colonized by a large number of microorganisms, at least 100 trillion of them, which maintain symbiotic relationships with the host [1] and contribute to various functions of the body,

Y. Ogawa (✉) · Y. Honda · T. Kessoku · W. Tomeno · K. Imajo · M. Yoneda · S. Saito
A. Nakajima
Department of Gastroenterology and Hepatology, Yokohama City University Graduate School of Medicine, Yokohama, Japan
e-mail: ogaway@yokohama-cu.ac.jp

H. Yoshiji, K. Kaji (eds.), *Alcoholic/Non-Alcoholic Digestive Diseases*,
https://doi.org/10.1007/978-981-13-1465-0_9

including digestion, vitamin synthesis, and resistance to colonization of the intestine by pathogens [2]. The number of species present increases from the esophagus to the rectum, ranging from 101/g of contents in the upper gastrointestinal tract to 1012/g of contents in the distal part of the intestine [3]. Its composition is strongly influenced by several factors, including environmental hygiene. The bacterial contents in the microbiota have been classified according to the phylum, order, family, genus, or species, in relative abundance values, and more than 90% of the microbiota belong to two phyla, namely, Firmicutes and Bacteroidetes, followed by Actinobacteria and Verrucomicrobia. Normal gut microbiota is considered to confer several physiologic benefits on the host, including immune system development, protection from pathogens, and regulation of intestinal homeostasis and metabolic functions. On the other hand, qualitative/quantitative alterations of the gut microbiota, called dysbiosis, are considered to predispose to the development and progression of several chronic liver diseases [2, 4–10].

9.2 NAFLD and Gut Microbiota

9.2.1 Dysbiosis

Ectopic accumulation of triglycerides in the liver, in the absence of other liver disease or a history of chronic alcohol consumption, is termed non-alcoholic fatty liver disease (NAFLD). It is estimated that NAFLD affects approximately 19% of the adult population, and that NAFLD is associated with the worldwide epidemic of metabolic syndrome, characterized by concurrent occurrence of obesity and insulin resistance [11]. Patients with NAFLD (non-alcoholic fatty liver [NAFL] and non-alcoholic steatohepatitis [NASH]) may eventually develop progressive liver fibrosis, with the risk of progression to cirrhosis and/or hepatocellular carcinoma (HCC). Evidence is increasing that the gut and liver show interdependence at multiple levels, and disturbance of the gut-liver axis has been implicated in the pathogenesis of a number of conditions linked to obesity, including NAFLD. Evidence also indicates that the microbial populations are altered in patients with NAFLD (Table 9.1) [2].

Dysbiosis can result from a wide range of environmental, immunological, and host factors, as well as from alterations of the bile flow, gastric pH, and/or intestinal dysmotility. In the case of fatty liver, early evidence linking gut dysbiosis to liver injury was obtained from descriptive human studies showing an association between NASH and small intestinal bacterial overgrowth as assessed by combined 14C D-xylose and lactulose breath testing [12]. Deficits in the mixing adequacy and transit time of gut contents can lead to bacterial overgrowth and nutrient malabsorption. In the case of short-chain fatty acids (SCFAs), malabsorption causes release of peptide YY (PYY) which slows gastric emptying and small intestinal transit [13]. The mixing adequacy and transit time are controlled by enteric neurons. A diet high

Table 9.1 Dysbiosis in NAFLD and PSC [2, 25]

Disease	Subject	Result			Study
NAFLD/NASH					
.	Human	phylum	Firmicutes		Raman M, et al. Clin Gastroenterol Hepatol 2013;11:868–875. e1–3
		genus	↑	*Oscillibacter*	
			↓	*Lactobacillus, Robinsoniella, Roseburia, Dorea*	
	Human	phylum	↑	Actinobacteria, Bacteroidetes, Proteobacteria	Boursier J, et al. Hepatology 2016;63:764–765
			↓	Firmicutes	
		genus	↑	*Parabacteroides, Prevotella, Sutterella*	
			↓	*Bifidobacterium, Bacteroidetes, Blautia, Ruminococcus*	
	Human	Phylum		Firmicutes, Proteobacteria	Bajaj JS, et al. J Hepatol 2014;60:940–947
		Family	↑	*Family XIV Incertae sedis, Lachnospiraceae, Ruminococcaceae*	
			↓	*Enterobacteriaceae, Holomonadaceae*	
	Human	Phylum	Bacteroidetes		Mutlu EA, et al. Am J Physiol Gastrointest Liver Physiol 2012;302:G966–G978
		Family	↑	*Bacteroidaceae*	
PSC					
	Human	genus	↑	*Veillonella*	Kummen et al. Gut. 2017; 66:611–619
	Human	genus	↑	*Escherichia, Lachnospiraceae, Megasphaera*	Quraishi et al. Gut 2017; 66: 386–388
			↓	*Prevotella, Roseburia*	

in fat, cholesterol, and fructose resulted in degeneration and loss of 15–30% of the enteric neurons and damage to the remaining neurons [14]. Wigg et al. found a higher prevalence of small intestinal bacterial overgrowth syndrome (SIBO) in patients with NASH as compared to healthy control subjects [12].

Thus, reduced gut motility, in which the nutrients are not adequately mixed and absorbed, could contribute to bacterial overgrowth, dysbiosis, and progression of steatohepatitis.

9.2.2 *Increased Intestinal Permeability*

The liver has both an arterial and venous blood supply, with the majority of the hepatic blood flow from the gut flowing via the portal vein. Therefore, it is exposed to potentially harmful substances derived from the gut, including translocated bacteria, lipopolysaccharides (LPS) or endotoxins, and secreted cytokines.

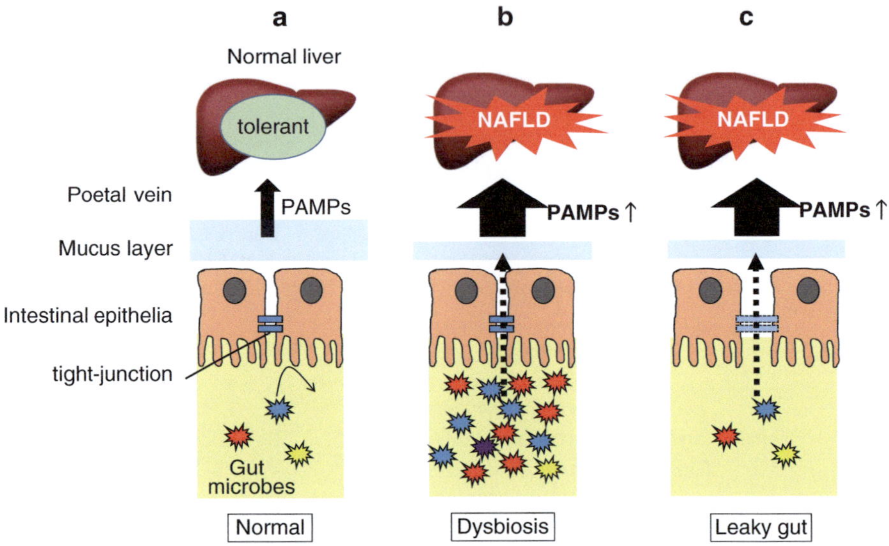

Fig. 9.1 Gut-liver axis. (**a**) The normal liver is relatively more tolerant to small amounts of PAMPs. (**b**) Changes in the composition of the intestinal bacterial flora increase the exposure of the liver to PAMPs to the liver via the portal vein. (**c**) Breakdown of the barrier function of the intestinal wall increases the exposure of the liver to PAMPs via the portal vein

Under physiological conditions, tight junction proteins, such as zonula occludens, seal the junctions between intestinal endothelial cells at their apical aspect, and thus have a vital role in preventing the translocation of harmful substances from the gut into the portal system. Dysbiosis can disrupt these tight junctions, increasing mucosal permeability and exposing both the gut mucosal cells and liver to potentially pro-inflammatory bacterial products (Fig. 9.1). For example, hepatic steatosis induced by a high-fat diet is associated with dysbiosis and increased intestinal permeability, with translocation of bacterial LPS from the gram-negative bacilli in the gut [15].

The immune system recognizes pathogen-associated molecular patterns (PAMPs) via pattern recognition receptors (PRRs), such as toll-like receptors (TLRs) and nucleotide-binding oligomerization domain-like receptors (NLR). TLRs are multiprotein complexes that recognize PAMPs, such as bacterial peptidoglycans or LPS, double-stranded DNA and RNA (dsDNA, dsRNA), and danger-associated molecular patterns. Activation of the TLR pathway is involved in inflammation and cell death [16].

9.2.3 Sensitivity of the Liver to Endotoxins

The term "metabolic endotoxemia" was coined when Cani et al. discovered that the microbiome is involved in the onset of insulin resistance, low-grade inflammation, and diabetes [17]. They found that metabolic endotoxemia also triggers liver fat accumulation [17]. This effect was abolished in mice lacking the LPS receptor complex CD14/TLR4 [17, 18], indicating a direct link between the gut microbiota and the development of hepatic steatosis. We demonstrated that upregulation of CD14 by obesity-induced leptin-mediated signaling is critical to the hyperresponsiveness of the liver to endotoxin during the progression of NASH (Fig. 9.2) [19].

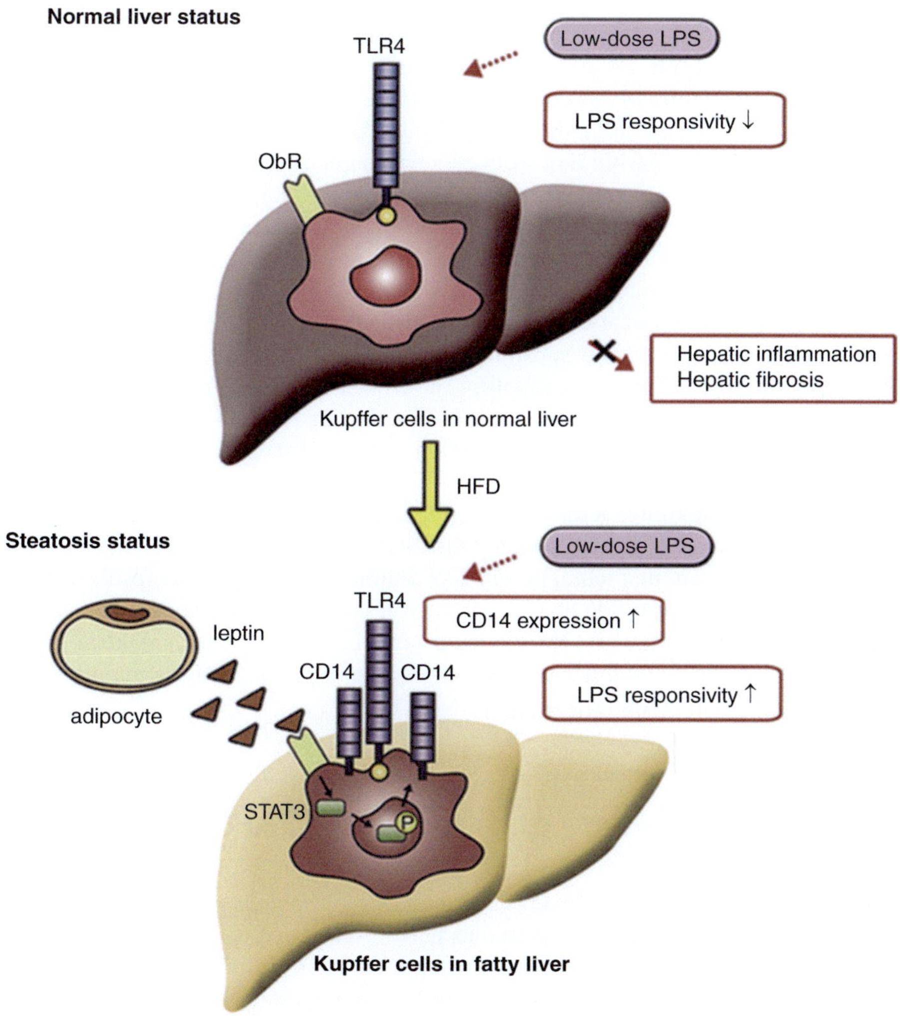

Fig. 9.2 HFD-induced steatosis in mice promotes hyperresponsiveness to low-dose LPS [19]. Upregulation of CD14 in the Kupffer cells and hyperresponsiveness to low-dose LPS were observed in a mouse model of high-fat diet (HFD)-induced steatosis, but not in the chow-fed control mice. Hyperresponsiveness to low-dose LPS led to accelerated NASH progression, including liver inflammation and fibrosis. Administration of leptin to chow-fed mice was associated with increased hepatic expression of CD14 via STAT3 signaling, resulting in hyperresponsiveness to low-dose LPS without steatosis

Thus, low-level endotoxin-mediated mechanism is important for the progression of NAFLD.

9.2.4 *Effects of Short-Chain Fatty Acids*

SCFAs, such as acetic, propionic, and butyric acids, are the major products of carbohydrate fermentation by gut microorganisms, with the normal gut microbiome producing 50–100 mmol/L/day of these compounds [20]. These SCFAs have effects on energy metabolism, immunity, and adipose tissue expansion. Many of these effects are mediated via binding to G-protein coupled receptors expressed in the immune system and on endocrine cells of the gut and adipocytes. The types and amounts of SCFAs synthesized in the gut vary with the amounts of carbohydrate compounds consumed and by dysbiosis, and there are multiple mechanisms through which they might contribute to the progression of NAFLD [5].

Butyrate and propionate can regulate intestinal physiology and immune functions, while acetate acts as a substrate for lipogenesis and gluconeogenesis [21]. Recently, key roles of these metabolites have been identified in the regulation of immune functions in the peripheral tissues, directing appropriate immune responses, oral tolerance and resolution of inflammation, and also for regulating the inflammatory output of adipose tissue [22].

Fermentation of amino acids, besides releasing beneficial SCFAs, also produces a range of potentially harmful compounds. Studies in animal models and in vitro studies have shown that compounds like ammonia, phenols, p-cresol, certain amines, and hydrogen sulfide play important roles in the initiation or progression of a leaky gut and inflammation [23]. On the contrary, dietary fiber and intake of plant-based foods appear to inhibit this, highlighting the importance of maintaining gut-microbiome carbohydrate fermentation [24].

9.3 Primary Sclerosing Cholangitis (PSC) and Gut Microbiota

PSC is encountered at a relatively high incidence in patients with inflammatory bowel disorder (IBD), and recent studies have investigated the gut microbiome in relation to the development of patients with PSC. PSC is presumed to be an autoimmune disorder, however, it is speculated that the gut microbiota is also relevant to its pathogenesis, in particular, because PSC is often associated with IBD and aberrant lymphocyte tracking, and significant gut-liver axes exist through bile acid signaling. It is likely that intestinal bacteria could trigger an abnormal or inadequate immune response that eventually leads to liver damage and fibrosis. Recently, patients with PSC have been shown to exhibit a distinct gut microbiota (Table 9.1) [25].

There is evidence that mucosal integrity is compromised in patients with PSC, supporting the traditional leaky gut hypothesis of microbe-derived products translocating to the liver and biliary system to trigger an inflammatory reactions [26].

These findings collectively suggest that bacterial antigens translocate across a leaky, and possibly inflamed, gut wall into the portal and biliary systems to elicit an abnormal immune response and trigger PSC pathogenesis.

9.4 Treatment

The gut-liver axis is widely implicated in the pathogenesis of liver diseases, and has increasingly been the focus of related clinical research. Recent trials of an array of therapeutic strategies have yielded promising results (Table 9.2) [10]. Bile acids and

Table 9.2 Ongoing clinical trials targeting the gut-liver axis [10]

Medication	Mechanism	Trial phase	Primary endpoint
NAFLD/NASH			
Solithromycin	Antibiotic	Phase II	Safety, NAFLD activity score in histology
Oligofructose-enriched inulin	Pre-biotic	–	Liver injury, fat, fibrosis
Oligofructose-enriched inulin	Pre-biotic	–	Liver fat, injury, inflammation
VSL3	Pro-biotic	–	NAFLD activity score at 1 year
Bio-25/subherb	Pro-biotic	–	Ultrasound liver fat
Lactobacillus acidophilus ATCC SD5221 and 1.109 Bifidobacterium lactis HN019	Pro-biotic	–	Liver biopsy 6 months
Lactobacillus spp.	Pro-biotic	–	Plasma LPS 12 weeks
Bifidobacterium animals/lactis + fructooligosaccharide	Symbiotic	–	Liver fat, insulin resistance
OCA	FXR-agonist	Phase III	Mortality, liver-related outcomes at 5-year FU
LJN452	FXR-agonist	Phase II	Safety, tolerability, AST, ALT
GS9674	FXR-agonist	Phase II	Safety, tolerability, AST, ALT
PX104	FXR-agonist	Phase II	Safety
SHP626 Volixibat	ASBT-inhibitor	Phase II	NAFLD-activity score
Aramchol	Fatty-acid bile acid compound	Phase II	% change in the liver triglycerides
NGM282	Recomb FGF19	Phase II	Liver fat content 12 weeks
BMS-986036	Recomb FGF21	Phase II	Safety, liver fat
PSC			
Flagyl or vancomycin	Antibiotic	Phase IV	Liver function test
Vancomycin	Antibiotic	Phase IV	Liver function test at 12 weeks
OCA	FXR-agonist	Phase II	Safety, AP, transaminases
GS9674	FXR-agonist	Phase II	Safety, tolerability
NGM282	Recomb FGF19	Phase II	Change in AP

the signaling pathways activated mainly via the nuclear FXR are key players in the gut-liver axis, affecting the intestinal barrier function, as well as lipid and glucose metabolism. Hence, multiple promising pharmacological FXR modulators are currently under trial for the treatment of NAFLD and various other liver diseases [10].

9.5 Conclusions

The gut microbiota contributes significantly to the onset and progression of liver diseases and influences the risk of complications in patients with end-stage liver disease. Future studies should assess the expression profiles of microbial genes, proteins, and metabolites, focusing especially on clinical patients. Increasing our understanding of the delicate homeostasis between the intestine and its microbiota could provide new insights into the pathogenesis of liver diseases and pave the way for the development of suitable therapeutic strategies.

References

1. Neish AS. Microbes in gastrointestinal health and disease. Gastroenterology. 2009;136:65–80.
2. Betrapally NS, Gillevet PM, Bajaj JS. Changes in the intestinal microbiome and alcoholic and nonalcoholic liver diseases: causes or effects? Gastroenterology. 2016;150:1745–1755.e1743.
3. Jandhyala SM, Talukdar R, Subramanyam C, Vuyyuru H, Sasikala M, Nageshwar Reddy D. Role of the normal gut microbiota. World J Gastroenterol. 2015;21:8787–803.
4. Gonzalez FJ, Jiang C, Patterson AD. An intestinal microbiota-farnesoid X receptor axis modulates metabolic disease. Gastroenterology. 2016;151:845–59.
5. Leung C, Rivera L, Furness JB, Angus PW. The role of the gut microbiota in NAFLD. Nat Rev Gastroenterol Hepatol. 2016;13:412–25.
6. Marchesi JR, Adams DH, Fava F, Hermes GD, Hirschfield GM, Hold G, Quraishi MN, et al. The gut microbiota and host health: a new clinical frontier. Gut. 2016;65:330–9.
7. Marra F, Svegliati-Baroni G. Lipotoxicity and the gut-liver axis in NASH pathogenesis. J Hepatol. 2018;68:280–95.
8. Schnabl B, Brenner DA. Interactions between the intestinal microbiome and liver diseases. Gastroenterology. 2014;146:1513–24.
9. Tilg H, Cani PD, Mayer EA. Gut microbiome and liver diseases. Gut. 2016;65:2035–44.
10. Wiest R, Albillos A, Trauner M, Bajaj JS, Jalan R. Targeting the gut-liver axis in liver disease. J Hepatol. 2017;67:1084–103.
11. Younossi ZM, Stepanova M, Negro F, Hallaji S, Younossi Y, Lam B, Srishord M. Nonalcoholic fatty liver disease in lean individuals in the United States. Medicine (Baltimore). 2012;91:319–27.
12. Wigg AJ, Roberts-Thomson IC, Dymock RB, McCarthy PJ, Grose RH, Cummins AG. The role of small intestinal bacterial overgrowth, intestinal permeability, endotoxaemia, and tumour necrosis factor alpha in the pathogenesis of non-alcoholic steatohepatitis. Gut. 2001;48:206–11.
13. Musso G, Gambino R, Cassader M. Obesity, diabetes, and gut microbiota: the hygiene hypothesis expanded? Diabetes Care. 2010;33:2277–84.

14. Rivera LR, Leung C, Pustovit RV, Hunne BL, Andrikopoulos S, Herath C, Testro A, et al. Damage to enteric neurons occurs in mice that develop fatty liver disease but not diabetes in response to a high-fat diet. Neurogastroenterol Motil. 2014;26:1188–99.
15. Saito T, Hayashida H, Furugen R. Comment on: Cani et al. (2007) Metabolic endotoxemia initiates obesity and insulin resistance: Diabetes 56:1761-1772. Diabetes. 2007;56:e20; author reply e21
16. Szabo G, Iracheta-Vellve A. Inflammasome activation in the liver: focus on alcoholic and non-alcoholic steatohepatitis. Clin Res Hepatol Gastroenterol. 2015;39(Suppl 1):S18–23.
17. Cani PD, Amar J, Iglesias MA, Poggi M, Knauf C, Bastelica D, Neyrinck AM, et al. Metabolic endotoxemia initiates obesity and insulin resistance. Diabetes. 2007;56:1761–72.
18. Cani PD, Bibiloni R, Knauf C, Waget A, Neyrinck AM, Delzenne NM, Burcelin R. Changes in gut microbiota control metabolic endotoxemia-induced inflammation in high-fat diet-induced obesity and diabetes in mice. Diabetes. 2008;57:1470–81.
19. Imajo K, Fujita K, Yoneda M, Nozaki Y, Ogawa Y, Shinohara Y, Kato S, et al. Hyperresponsivity to low-dose endotoxin during progression to nonalcoholic steatohepatitis is regulated by leptin-mediated signaling. Cell Metab. 2012;16:44–54.
20. Duncan SH, Louis P, Thomson JM, Flint HJ. The role of pH in determining the species composition of the human colonic microbiota. Environ Microbiol. 2009;11:2112–22.
21. Macfarlane GT, Macfarlane S. Fermentation in the human large intestine: its physiologic consequences and the potential contribution of prebiotics. J Clin Gastroenterol. 2011;45(Suppl):S120–7.
22. Arpaia N, Campbell C, Fan X, Dikiy S, van der Veeken J, deRoos P, Liu H, et al. Metabolites produced by commensal bacteria promote peripheral regulatory T-cell generation. Nature. 2013;504:451–5.
23. Windey K, de Preter V, Verbeke K. Relevance of protein fermentation to gut health. Mol Nutr Food Res. 2012;56:184–96.
24. Tang WH, Wang Z, Levison BS, Koeth RA, Britt EB, Fu X, Wu Y, et al. Intestinal microbial metabolism of phosphatidylcholine and cardiovascular risk. N Engl J Med. 2013;368:1575–84.
25. Quraishi MN, Sergeant M, Kay G, Iqbal T, Chan J, Constantinidou C, Trivedi P, et al. The gut-adherent microbiota of PSC-IBD is distinct to that of IBD. Gut. 2017;66:386–8.
26. Bjornsson E, Cederborg A, Akvist A, Simren M, Stotzer PO, Bjarnason I. Intestinal permeability and bacterial growth of the small bowel in patients with primary sclerosing cholangitis. Scand J Gastroenterol. 2005;40:1090–4.

Chapter 10
Role of Oxidative Stress in Alcoholic/Non-Alcoholic Liver Diseases

Keisuke Hino

Abstract Oxidative stress is the shift in the balance between oxidants and antioxidants in favor of oxidants. Reactive oxygen species (ROS) play a central role in inducing oxidative stress. Mitochondria are the main site of cellular ROS production, and simultaneously have a well-organized antioxidant system. Therefore, mitochondria have evolved multiple systems of quality control to ensure that the requisite number of functional mitochondria is present to meet the demands of the cell. The liver also is the major iron storage organ in the body and therefore mild to moderate degrees of hepatic iron accumulation are sometimes involved in chronic liver diseases. Iron overload, especially excess divalent iron can be highly toxic, mainly via the Fenton reaction producing hydroxyl radicals. The liver is often a target of injury by oxidative stress. Oxidative stress has been shown to be present in alcoholic liver diseases, non-alcoholic steatohepatitis, and chronic hepatitis C to a greater degree than in other inflammatory liver diseases. This chapter highlights iron overload in the liver and mitochondrial ROS production through reduced mitochondrial quality control as important causative factors for inducing oxidative stress in chronic liver diseases, especially focusing on alcoholic liver disease, non-alcoholic steatohepatitis, and chronic hepatitis C.

Keywords Reactive oxygen species · Iron · Mitochondria · Mitochondria quality control · Non-alcoholic steatohepatitis · Chronic hepatitis C

10.1 Introduction

Reactive oxygen species (ROS) are produced by living organisms as a result of normal cellular metabolism and environmental factors. ROS are highly reactive molecules and can damage cell structures such as carbohydrates, nucleic acids,

K. Hino (✉)
Department of Hepatology and Pancreatology, Kawasaki Medical School, Kurashiki, Okayama, Japan
e-mail: khino@med.kawasaki-m.ac.jp

H. Yoshiji, K. Kaji (eds.), *Alcoholic/Non-Alcoholic Digestive Diseases*,
https://doi.org/10.1007/978-981-13-1465-0_10

lipids, and proteins and alter their functions. However, since the body is able to remove ROS to a certain degree, these reactive species are not necessarily a threat to the body under physiological conditions [1, 2]. ROS are required at a certain level in the body to perform its important physiological functions. The shift in the balance between oxidants and antioxidants in favor of oxidants is termed "oxidative stress." Oxidative stress contributes to many pathological conditions and diseases. The liver is often a target of injury by oxidative stress. Many risk factors, including alcohol, drugs, environmental pollutants, and irradiation, may induce oxidative stress in the liver, which in turn results in severe liver diseases. Oxidative stress has been shown to be present in alcoholic liver disease, non-alcoholic steatohepatitis (NASH), and chronic hepatitis C to a greater degree than in other inflammatory liver diseases. Interestingly, these diseases have iron overload and mitochondrial injury in the liver in common. This chapter will review and discuss the role of oxidative stress in liver diseases, especially focusing on hepatic iron overload and mitochondrial ROS production.

10.2 Oxidative Stress in the Liver

In mammals, an organized antioxidant system has developed to maintain the redox homeostasis in the liver. Both enzymatic and non-enzymatic antioxidant systems are essential for cellular responses in order to deal with oxidative stress under physiological conditions. Antioxidant enzymes such as catalase, superoxide dismutase (SOD), and glutathione peroxidase and non-enzymatic electron receptors such as glutathione (GSH) are affected and used as indexes to evaluate the level of oxidative stress [3]. Erythroid 2-related factor 2 (Nrf2) is a major regulator of cellular redox balance [3, 4]. Nrf2 physiologically binds to kelch-like ECH-associated protein-1 (Keap1) in the cytoplasm, and is inactivated and easily degraded. Under oxidative stress Nrf2 dissociates from Keap1 via Keap1 modification or Nrf2 phosphorylation and is activated. The activated Nrf2 translocates into the nucleus and interacts with the antioxidant response element, promoting the expression of cytoprotective target genes, including antioxidant enzymes and phase II detoxifying enzymes [3, 5–7].

When there are excessive ROS, the homeostasis is disturbed, resulting in oxidative stress, which plays a critical role in liver diseases and other chronic and degenerative disorders. This oxidative stress triggers hepatic damage by inducing alterations of lipids, proteins, and DNA contents and modulating pathways that control normal biological functions. Since these pathways regulate the transcription of genes, protein expression, cell apoptosis, and hepatic stellate cell activation, oxidative stress is considered to be a pathological mechanism that results in the initiation and progression of various liver diseases, such as alcoholic liver disease, NASH, and chronic viral hepatitis [3].

10.3 Iron and Oxidative Stress in Liver Diseases

The liver is the major iron storage organ in the body and therefore mild to moderate degrees of hepatic iron accumulation are sometimes involved in chronic liver diseases [8–12]. Iron overload, especially excess divalent iron can be highly toxic, mainly via the Fenton reaction producing hydroxyl radicals [13]. This is particularly relevant for liver diseases with mild to moderate iron overloaded such as alcoholic liver disease, NASH, and chronic hepatitis C, in which oxidative stress has been proposed to be a major mechanism of liver injury. Oxidative stress and increased iron levels strongly favor DNA damage, genetic instability, and tumorigenesis. Indeed, a significant correlation between 8-hydroxy-2′-deoxyguanosine (8-OHdG), a marker of oxidatively generated DNA damage [14] and hepatic iron excess has been shown in iron overloaded liver diseases.

10.3.1 Iron Overload in Alcohol Liver Disease

Patients with alcoholic liver disease frequently exhibit iron overload in association with increased hepatic fibrosis. Even moderate alcohol consumption elevates body iron stores. Hepcidin, a 25 amino-acid peptide synthesized in the liver, is a key mediator of iron metabolism, and acts to attenuate both intestinal iron absorption and iron release from reticuloendothelial macrophages [15, 16]. As one of the mechanisms underlying alcohol-induced iron overload, alcohol metabolism-mediated oxidative stress has been shown to regulate hepcidin transcription via a transcription factor, CCAAT/enhancer-binding protein α (C/EBPα), which in turn leads to increased duodenal iron transport [17].

When hepatocytes accumulates excess iron in clinical alcohol abuse or in an experimental model of combined iron and alcohol hepatotoxity, there is evidence for synergy among the putative pathways of oxidative stress. How excess hepatocytic iron accumulates in alcoholic excess is unknown, but when the usual safe harbor for intracellular iron, namely the endosomal-lysosomal compartment, is compromised, it becomes a potent source of free, chelatable pro-oxidant iron. In this regard excess iron in alcohol-induced liver damage and alcohol excess in iron overload disease are powerful cocktails promoting subcellular organelle damage leading to cell death and fibrogenesis [18].

10.3.2 Iron Overload in NASH

Non-alcoholic fatty liver disease (NAFLD) is present in 10–30% of the world's population. A recent large cohort study showed that 35% of subjects enrolled in the NASH Clinical Research Network had stainable hepatic iron [19]. In animal models of fatty liver, iron loading is associated with the development of hepatic inflammation and fibrosis [20]. Early reports on the association of hepatic iron with NAFLD and NASH were controversial. However, more recent studies have strongly suggested a causative role for iron in the development of NASH, demonstrating that increased hepatic iron contributes to progression of NAFLD [9, 21]. In addition to the induction of oxidative stress, iron has been implicated as a cofactor in the pathogenesis of insulin resistance, which is universal among individuals with NAFLD and is implicated in the progression of liver injury [22]. Iron also appears to be a risk factor for the development of HCC in patients with NASH. Iron overload in patients with NASH-related cirrhosis is reported to be potentially associated with HCC development [23].

The precise mechanisms by which some patients with NASH are prone to hepatic iron accumulation remain elusive. However, several mechanisms have been proposed (Table 10.1). Aigner et al. suggested an impaired release of iron from liver cells as an underlying mechanism for iron accumulation in NAFLD [32]. They found down-regulation of the *ferroportin-1* and *hemojuvelin* (*Hjv*) genes, probably due to an increase in tumor necrosis-alpha (TFN-α). This also explains the characteristic pattern of iron deposition in NAFLD, which is different from the pattern seen in hereditary hemochromatosis; i.e., hepatic and sinusoidal deposition without a zonal gradient. Transgenic mice expressing the retinoic acid receptor alpha-dominant

Table 10.1 Proposed mechanisms by which hepatic iron accumulates in NAFLD/NASH

Factor(s) related to iron metabolic disorders	Intermediary molecules	Molecules responsible for iron accumulation	Affected pathway in iron transport	References
Increased TNF-α[a] production	Hemojuvelin	Ferroportin-1	Iron release from hepatocytes and Kupffer cells	[24]
Impaired retinoic acid signaling	Hemojuvelin, TfR2[b]	Ferroportin-1	Iron release from hepatocytes and Kupffer cells	[25, 26]
Erythrocytes		Phosphatidylserine	Erythrocyte phagocytosis by Kupffer cells	[27]
Undetermined humoral factor(s)	IRP1	Dmt1[c]	Duodenal iron absorption	[28]
Copper deficiency	Ceruloplasmin	Ferroportin-1	Iron release from hepatocytes and Kupffer cells	[29]
ROS[d] production	Ceruloplasmin	Ferroportin-1	Iron release from hepatocytes and Kupffer cells	[30]

Adopted from Table 7.1 in "The Liver in Systemic Diseases" edited by Ohira H [31]
[a]Tumor necrosis factor alpha
[b]Transferrin receptor 2
[c]Divalent metal transporter
[d]Reactive oxygen species

negative form in hepatocytes develop steatohepatitis and liver tumors [24]. Hepatic iron accumulates in these mice, and retinoid treatment decreases hepatic iron content through suppression of Hjv expression [25]. These results suggest that impaired retinoic acid function is responsible for hepatic iron accumulation in NASH. Otogawa et al. indicated that the engulfment of phosphatidylserine-externalized, apoptotic signal-positive erythrocytes by hepatic macrophages might lead to the accumulation of iron derived from hemoglobin in the liver of NASH [26]. Interestingly, a recent study has demonstrated that duodenal iron absorption increases through upregulation of Dmt1, regardless of elevation of the serum Hepcidin level in patients with NASH [27]. Undetermined humoral factor(s) contained in sera of NASH patients activated IRP1, which subsequently up-regulates Dmt1 expression through the IRP/IRE system [27].

Iron accumulation may be linked to copper homeostasis. One study reported that copper status was linked to iron homeostasis in NAFLD, suggesting that low copper bioavailability causes increased hepatic iron stores via decreased ferroportin-1 expression and ceruloplasmin ferroxidase activity, thus blocking liver iron export in copper-deficient subjects [28]. In addition, oxidative stress/ROS in hepatic cells has been demonstrated to down-regulate ceruloplasmin via a novel mRNA decay mechanism that may contribute to hepatic iron accumulation by decreasing hepatic iron release [29].

10.3.3 Iron Overload in Chronic Hepatitis C

Based on the assumption that one-third of iron stores are normally in the liver, this would translate to a normal median hepatic iron content of 0.27 g for men and 0.13 g for women [30]. Extensive studies reported median hepatic iron concentrations of 396 [range: 0–2105] and 458 [range: 114–2190] μg/g dry weight liver tissue in patients with chronic hepatitis C [33, 34]. These results suggest that the hepatic iron content in patients with chronic hepatitis C is approximately 0.50–0.69 g, equivalent to 2–5 times the normal hepatic iron content if the liver weight is estimated to be 1500 g.

The role of *HFE* mutations in chronic hepatitis C has been well reviewed [35]. In general, patients with chronic hepatitis C seem to have no difference in the prevalence of heterozygosity for *HFE* mutations as compared with a control population. The levels of hepatic hepcidin mRNA and serum Hepcidin, that is, the 25 amino acid bioactive hepcidin, are reported to be lower in in patients with chronic hepatitis C than in those with chronic hepatitis B or controls despite a significant correlation between hepcidin and serum ferritin or the histological iron score in both groups [36, 37]. Thus, the relatively decreased synthesis of hepcidin in chronic hepatitis C contrasts with the absolute deficit or lack of hepcidin synthesis observed in hereditary hemochromatosis and may account for the mild to moderate hepatic iron overload observed in some patients with chronic hepatitis C. The mechanisms underlying hepatitis C virus (HCV)-related hepatic iron overload appear to have some similarities with alcohol-induced iron overload in terms of disrupted hepcidin transcription through suppressed activity of C/EBPα due to ROS [17, 38].

Hepcidin is potentially regulated through the bone morphogenic protein (BMP)/sons of mothers against decapentaplegic (SMAD) cascade by both circulating transferrin-bound iron and intracellular iron stores in chronic hepatitis C. Taking into account the significant correlation between hepcidin expression and serum ferritin or the histological iron score [36, 37], hepcidin transcription seems to be properly regulated in response to the iron concentration in chronic hepatitis C. Thus, the opposing effects of HCV-induced hepcidin-suppressive factors and iron-load-induced hepcidin-stimulation factors potentially regulate hepcidin transcription in chronic hepatitis C. Inflammation also regulates hepcidin transcription. Proinflammatory cytokines such as IL-6 mediate this response by inducing transcription of hepcidin mRNA via signal transducer and activator of transcription (STAT)3, which binds to a STAT-responsive element within the hepcidin promoter [39]. Serum levels of IL-6 have been shown to be elevated in patients with HCV-related chronic liver disease [40], which raises the possibility that IL-6 acts to stimulate hepcidin expression through the STAT3 pathway. This would be expected to counteract the decrease in hepcidin transcription caused by HCV-induced ROS. On the other hand, chronic inflammation with production of proinflammatory cytokines has the potential to deliver an additional burden of ROS, which would be expected to reinforce the decrease in hepcidin transcription. Most likely, during chronic inflammation states in vivo like chronic hepatitis C, the regulation of hepcidin is more complex and may depend on many variables, including the particular stage of systemic and/or hepatic inflammatory disease. This might explain the variations in hepatic iron concentrations reported among patients with HCV-related chronic liver disease. The schematic outline in Fig. 10.1 depicts the assumed mechanisms underlying the hepatic iron accumulation in chronic hepatitis C.

10.4 Mitochondria-Derived Oxidative Stress

The mitochondrial electron transport system consists of several multipolypeptide protein complexes (I-V) embedded in the inner mitochondrial membrane that receive electrons from reducing equivalents (i.e., nicotinamide adenine dinucleotide [NADH] and flavin adenine dinucleotide [$FADH_2$]) generated by dehydrogenases (e.g., pyruvate dehydrogenase, α-ketoglutarate dehydrogenase, acyl-CoA dehydrogenase, etc.). These electrons flow through the complex I, the ubiquinone cycle (Q/QH_2), complex III, cytochrome c, complex IV, and to the final acceptor O_2 to form H_2O. Electron flow through complexes I, III, and IV results in the pumping of protons to the outer surface of the inner membrane, establishing a membrane potential that is used by adenosine triphosphate (ATP) synthetase to drive the rephosphorylation of ADP. Several of the redox couples within the electron transport chain transfer single rather than two electrons and are therefore susceptible to leaking electrons directly to surrounding O_2 to form the free-radical superoxide ($O_2^{\bullet -}$).

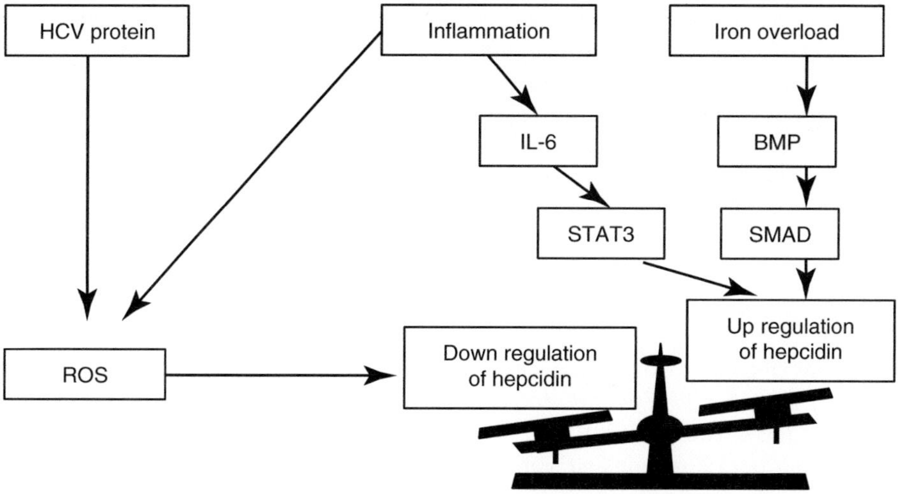

Fig. 10.1 Schematic diagram depicting the assumed mechanisms underlying the hepatic iron accumulation in patients with chronic hepatitis C. Hepcidin transcription in chronic hepatitis C may be potentially regulated by the opposing effects of HCV-related ROS-induced hepcidin suppression and iron load-induced hepcidin stimulation. Inflammation may also have the opposing effects of stimulation and suppression of hepcidin transcription through the IL-6/STAT pathway and ROS pathway, respectively. Consequent relative suppression of hepcidin expression is potentially one of the mechanisms underlying the hepatic iron accumulation in patients with chronic hepatitis C. *HCV* hepatitis C virus, *ROS* reactive oxygen species, *IL-6* interleukin 6, *STAT* signal transducer and activator of transcription, *BMP* bone morphogenic protein, *SMAD* sons of mothers against decapentaplegic. Adopted from Fig. 7.1 in "The Liver in Systemic Diseases" edited by Ohira H [31]

The detoxification of ROS is an important function of the cellular redox homeostasis system. Cells rapidly convert $O_2^{\bullet-}$ into the two-electron nonradical hydrogen peroxide (H_2O_2) via manganese SOD (MnSOD). H_2O_2 in turn can be further reduced to H_2O in the mitochondrial matrix by GSH or the thioredoxin/peroxiredoxin systems, or can freely diffuse out of the mitochondria where it again is buffered by GSH [41].

10.4.1 ROS Production in Alcoholic Liver Disease

Alcohol metabolism occurs mainly in the liver, and alcohol is metabolized via both oxidative and non-oxidative pathways. Oxidative pathways are the predominant mechanism for alcohol metabolism. The most common pathway for oxidative metabolism in the liver is characterized by alcohol dehydrogenase (ADH), which metabolizes alcohol into acetaldehyde. Alcohol can also be oxidized into acetaldehyde by cytochrome P450 2E1 (CYP2E1) and catalase. Acetaldehyde is further metabolized into acetate and acetyl-CoA for use in metabolic pathways by aldehyde dehydrogenase (ALDH), which has two isoforms: cytosolic ALDH1 and mitochondrial ALDH2 [42]. The deleterious ethanol-mediated effects have been largely attributed to ethanol-induced oxidative stress and the subsequent damaging effects on mitochondria and other cellular compartments. ROS-producing proteins causing ethanol-mediated tissue injury include CYP2E1, inducible nitric oxide synthase (iNOS), nicotinamide adenine dinucleotide phosphate (NADPH) oxidase, xanthine oxidase, and mitochondrial complexes [43]. CYP2E1 is indeed suggested to induce its damaging effects in the liver following ethanol exposure due to its ability to produce oxidative radicals such as hydrogen peroxide and superoxide anions. There are several lines of evidence to support the location of CYP2E1 not only in endoplasmic reticulum but also in the mitochondria in vivo and in vitro. Direct damage of mitochondrial DNA by oxidative radicals and/or post-translational protein modifications of many mitochondrial proteins largely contributes to the oxidative stress-mediated hepatic injury. Thus, CYP2E1 plays direct and/or permissive roles in promoting mitochondrial dysfunction and hepatotoxity.

10.4.2 ROS Production in NAFLD

In the setting of obesity and hepatic insulin resistance, the existing nutrient and hormonal milieu is altered, favoring increased hepatic triglyceride accumulation [44, 45]. In this environment, ectopic fat accumulation in the liver seems secondary to chronic free fatty acid overload from insulin-resistant, dysfunctional adipose tissue, together with higher rates of hepatic de novo lipogenesis [45], and is often associated with hepatic insulin resistance and hepatocyte death. Recent evidence suggests that continuous adaptation or remodeling of mitochondrial energetics, gene expression, morphology, and content play a key role in the pathogenesis of simple steatosis/NASH [46, 47]. Mitochondrial oxidative energetics encompasses multiple pathways that include β-oxidation, hepatic tricarboxylic acid (TCA) cycle, ketogenesis, respiratory chain activity, and ATP synthesis, all of which work in concert to maintain cellular homeostasis. These multiple pathways have been reported to be induced in several mouse models of nutritional overload, as well as in human subjects, when obesity and simple steatosis are present [48]. As generation of acetyl-CoA through β-oxidation and its terminal oxidation through the hepatic TCA cycle are major sources of energy generation, induction of TCA cycle flux could be obligatory for high energy-demanding processes (e.g., gluconeogenesis and lipogenesis) during states of substrate overload, including simple steatosis or NASH in obesity or type 2 diabetes mellitus. However, sustained induction of TCA cycle flux, and its uncoupling from mitochondrial respiration and ATP synthesis, may bring about the unwanted effect of fueling ROS generation and the development of tissue inflammation [48]. Indeed, defects in mitochondrial morphology, the electron transport chain, and ATP production have been documented in NAFLD along with high levels of ROS and other mediators of inflammation. Satapati et al. illustrated how a modest elevation of free fatty acid delivery into normal liver was enough to upregulate the mitochondrial oxidative machinery [49]. During obesity and hepatic insulin resistance, chronic free fatty acid overload and the sustained induction of mitochondrial TCA cycle flux can act as a metabolic mechanism that hastens oxidative stress, inflammation, and progression to NASH.

10.4.3 ROS Production in Chronic Hepatitis C

Schwer et al. have demonstrated that HCV core protein associates with the mitochondria-associated membrane (MAM) fraction, a point of close contact between the endoplasmic reticulum and mitochondrion [50]. Direct interaction of HCV core protein with mitochondria potentially modifies mitochondrial ROS production and scavenging, subsequently inducing oxidative stress. When mitochondrial electron transport activity is inhibited by HCV core protein [51, 52], electrons are likely to leak from the electron transport chain transfer, accelerating mitochondrial $O_2^{\bullet-}$ production and/or H_2O_2 emission.

Although sufficient intraorganelle Ca^{2+} concentrations are required to stimulate metabolism by activating enzymes critical for maintenance of the TCA cycle, prolonged increases of Ca^{2+} can, in turn, interfere with the activities of these enzymes. The TCA cycle activity affects the electron transport chain activity, which in turn affects the mitochondrial membrane potential. Thus, increased Ca^{2+} influx into mitochondria induces a substrate imbalance of the TCA cycle that leads to the generation of mitochondrial ROS, probably through the inhibition of electron transport chain activity. There are several lines of evidence indicating that HCV increases mitochondrial ROS production by modulating calcium signaling. HCV core protein enhances mitochondrial Ca^{2+} uptake in response to ER Ca^{2+} release through activation of the mitochondrial Ca^{2+} uniporter, which leads to increased mitochondrial ROS production [53, 54].

10.5 Mitochondrial Quality Control as a Therapeutic Option

The role of mitochondria in energy production sensitizes them to damage owing to exposure to high levels of ROS, a by-product of energy generation that can disturb protein folding and structures and cause mitochondrial DNA mutations. Thus, the mitochondria are targets for ROS and ROS generators. Therefore, mitochondria have evolved multiple systems of quality control to ensure that the requisite number of functional mitochondria is present to meet the demands of the cell. These pathways work to eliminate damaged mitochondrial proteins or parts of the mitochondrial network via mitochondria-specific autophagy (mitophagy) and renew components by adding proteins and lipids through biogenesis, collectively resulting in mitochondrial turnover [55].

Removing damaged mitochondria by mitophagy is a protective mechanism against alcohol-induced liver injury and steatosis because it serves to maintain a healthy population of mitochondria, which prevents cell death by reducing oxidative stress and preserving respiratory chain function and mitochondrial bioenergetics for efficient energy production. Alcohol metabolism produces ROS in the liver, and mitochondria damaged by ROS release pro-apoptotic proteins. Therefore, removal of these damaged mitochondria is necessary to reduce hepatocellular death and liver injury caused by heavy alcohol consumption [42, 56].

Chronic persistence of hepatic lipid overload leads to liver injury with inflammation, cell death, and fibrosis characteristic of NASH. Some alterations in lipid metabolism are at the level of lipid mobilization, because hepatic-autophagy related protein (ATG)7 deletion decreases triglyceride break down, resulting in lipid droplet accumulation. Failure of mitochondrial quality control because of their reduced turnover through mitophagy can promote oxidative stress through ROS production and activation of downstream inflammatory pathways. The combination of lipotoxicity, oxidative stress, and chronic activation of the inflammatory response upon autophagy failure often leads to hepatocyte cell death, thus recapitulating the hallmarks of NASH (inflammation, oxidative stress, cell death, and fibrosis) [57].

As mentioned above, HCV increases mitochondrial ROS production via direct interaction of HCV proteins with mitochondria and/or modulation of mitochondrial calcium signaling. The detoxification of ROS is an important function of the cellular redox homeostasis system. Under resting cellular conditions, the intracellular redox environment is in a relatively reduced state [58]. The question is how HCV-induced mitochondrial ROS production and the subsequent oxidative stress persist in spite of ROS-detoxifying agents such as MnSOD and/or GSH or the thioredoxin/peroxiredoxin systems. Reduction of mitophagy/autophagy at least partially accounts for persistent ROS production in HCV infection because there are several lines of evidence that HCV infection suppresses autophagy flux at the step of fusion with lysosomes [59] or mitophagy by interacting with Parkin [60]. Thus, mitochondria quality control can be one of therapeutic strategies for alcoholic liver disease, NAFLD/NASH, and chronic hepatitis C.

10.6 Conclusion

Emerging evidence clearly illustrates the critical role of oxidative stress in the pathogenesis of chronic liver diseases such as alcoholic liver disease, NAFLD/NASH, and chronic hepatitis C. In this chapter, iron overload in the liver and mitochondrial ROS production through reduced mitochondrial quality control were highlighted as important causative factors for inducing oxidative stress in chronic liver diseases. Considering the robust relationship between iron overload, increased ROS production and oxidative stress in liver diseases, future studies should focus on the potential of promising therapeutic agents to attenuate iron overload and mitochondrial oxidative dysfunction.

References

1. McCord JM. The evolution of free radicals and oxidative stress. Am J Med. 2000;108:652–9.
2. Mittler R. Oxidative stress, antioxidants and stress tolerance. Trends Plant Sci. 2002;7:505–10.
3. Sha L, Tan HY, Wang N, et al. The role of oxidative stress and antioxidants in liver disease. Int J Mol Sci. 2015;16:26087–124.
4. Itoh K, Igarashi K, Hayashi N, et al. Cloning and characterization of a novel erythroid cell-derived CNC family transcription factor heterodimerizing with the small Maf family proteins. Mol Cell Biol. 1995;15:4184–93.
5. Kobayashi A, Kang MI, Okawa H, et al. Oxidative stress sensor Keap1 functions as an adaptor for Cul3-based E3 ligase to regulate proreosomal degradation of Nrf2. Mol Cell Biol. 2004;24:7130–9.
6. Kobayashi A, kang MI, Watai Y, et al. Oxidative and electrophilic stresses activate Nrf2 through inhibition of ubiquitination activity of Keap1. Mol Cell Biol. 2006;26:221–9.
7. Wakabayashi N, Itoh K, Wakabayashi J, et al. keap1-null mutation leads to postnatal lethality due to constitutive NRf2 activation. Nat Genet. 2003;35:238–45.
8. Peterson DR. Alcohol, iron-associated oxidative stress, and cancer. Alcohol. 2005;35:243–9.
9. George DK, Goldwurm S, MacDonald GA, et al. Increased hepatic iron concentration in nonalcoholic steatohepatitis is associated with increased fibrosis. Gastroenterology. 1998;114:311–8.
10. Sumida Y, Nakashima T, Yoh T, et al. Serum thioredoxin levels as a predictor of steatohepatitis in patients with nonalcoholic fatty liver disease. J Hepatol. 2003;38:32–8.
11. Farinati F, Cardin R, De Maria N, et al. Iron storage, lipid peroxidation and glutathione turnover in chronic anti-HCV positive hepatitis. J Hepatol. 1995;22:449–56.
12. di Bisceglie AM, Axiotis CA, Hoofnagle JH, Bacon BR. Measurements of iron status in patients with chronic hepatitis. Gastroenterology. 1992;102:2108–13.
13. Fenton HJH. Oxidation of tartaric acid in presence of iron. J Chem Soc. 1894;65:899–910.
14. Shibutani S, Takeshita M, Grollman AP. Insertion of specific bases during DNA synthesis past the oxidation-damaged base 8-oxodG. Nature. 1991;349:431–4.
15. Park CH, Valore EV, Waring AJ, Ganz T. Hepcidin, a urinary antimicrobial peptide synthesized in the liver. J Biol Chem. 2001;276:7806–10.
16. Ganz T. Hepcidin, a key regulator of iron metabolism and mediator of anemia of inflammation. Blood. 2003;102:783–8.
17. Harrison-Findik DD, Schafer D, Klein E, et al. Alcohol metabolism-mediated oxidative stress down-regulates hepcidin transcription and leads to increased duodenal iron transporter expression. J Biol Chem. 2006;281:22974–82.
18. Tavill AS, Qadri AM. Alcohol and iron. Semin Liver Dis. 2004;24:317–25.
19. Nelson JE, Wilson L, Brunt EM, et al. Relationship between the pattern of hepatic iron deposition and histological severity in nonalcoholic fatty liver disease. Hepatology. 2011;53:448–57.
20. Imeryuz N, Tahan V, Sonsuz A, et al. Iron preloading aggravates nutritional steatohepatitis in rats by increasing apoptotic cell death. J Hepatol. 2007;47:851–9.
21. Nelson JE, Bhattacharya R, Lindor KD, et al. HFE C282Y mutations are associated with advanced hepatic fibrosis in Caucasians with nonalcoholic steatohepatitis. Hepatology. 2007;46:723–9.
22. Smith BW, Adams LA. Nonalcoholic fatty liver disease and diabetes mellitus: pathogenesis and treatment. Nat Rev Endocrinol. 2011;7:456–65.
23. Sorrentino P, D'Angelo S, Ferbo U, Micheli P, Bracigliano A, Vecchione R. Liver iron excess in patients with hepatocellular carcinoma developed on non-alcoholic steato-hepatitis. J Hepatol. 2009;50:351–7.
24. Yanagitani A, Yamada S, Yasui S, et al. Retinoic acid receptor alpha dominant negative form causes steatohepatitis and liver tumors in transgenic mice. Hepatology. 2004;40:366–75.
25. Tsuchiya H, Akechi Y, Ikeda R, et al. Suppressive effects of retinoids on iron-induced oxidative stress in the liver. Gastroenterology. 2009;136:341–350 e8.

26. Otogawa K, Kinoshita K, Fujii H, et al. Erythrophagocytosis by liver macrophages (Kupffer cells) promotes oxidative stress, inflammation, and fibrosis in a rabbit model of steatohepatitis: implications for the pathogenesis of human nonalcoholic steatohepatitis. Am J Pathol. 2007;170:967–80.
27. Hoki T, Miyanishi K, Tanaka S, et al. Increased duodenal iron absorption through upregulation of divalent metal transporter 1 from enhancement of iron regulatory protein 1 activity in patients with nonalcoholic steatohepatitis. Hepatology. 2015;62:751–61.
28. Aigner E, Theurl I, Haufe H, et al. Copper availability contributes to iron perturbations in human nonalcoholic fatty liver disease. Gastroenterology. 2008;135:680–8.
29. Tapryal N, Mukhopadhyay C, Das D, Fox PL, Mukhopadhyay CK. Reactive oxygen species regulate ceruloplasmin by a novel mRNA decay mechanism involving its 3′-untranslated region: implications in neurodegenerative diseases. J Biol Chem. 2009;284:1873–83.
30. Rouault TA, Gordeuk V, Anderson G. The central role of the liver in iron storage and regulation of systemic iron homeostasis. In: Arias IM, et al., editors. The liver: biology and pathobiology. 5th ed. Hoboken: Wiley-Blackwell; 2009. p. 235–50.
31. Hino K, Harada M. Metal metabolism and liver. In: Ohira H, editor. The liver in systemic diseases. Heidelberg: Springer; 2016. p. 123–33.
32. Aigner E, Theurl I, Theurl M, et al. Pathways underlying iron accumulation in human nonalcoholic fatty liver disease. Am J Clin Nutr. 2008;87:1374–83.
33. Hofer H, Osterreicher C, Jessner W, et al. Hepatic iron concentration does not predict response to standard and pegylated-IFN/ribavirin therapy in patients with chronic hepatitis C. J Hepatol. 2004;40:1018–22.
34. Rulyak SJ, Eng SC, Patel K, McHutchison JG, Gordon SC, Kowdley KV. Relationships between hepatic iron content and virologic response in chronic hepatitis C patients treated with interferon and ribavirin. Am J Gastroenterol. 2005;100:332–7.
35. Pietrangelo A. Hemochromatosis gene modifies course of hepatitis C viral infection. Gastroenterology. 2003;124:1509–23.
36. Fujita N, Sugimoto R, Takeo M, et al. Hepcidin expression in the liver: relatively low level in patients with chronic hepatitis C. Mol Med. 2007;13:97–104.
37. Girelli D, Pasino M, Goodnough JB, et al. Reduced serum hepcidin levels in patients with chronic hepatitis C. J Hepatol. 2009;51:845–52.
38. Nishina S, Hino K, Korenaga M, et al. Hepatitis C virus-induced reactive oxygen species raise hepatic iron level in mice by reducing hepcidin transcription. Gastroenterology. 2008;134:226–38.
39. Pietrangelo A, Dierssen U, Valli L, et al. STAT3 is required for IL-6-gp130-dependent activation of hepcidin in vivo. Gastroenterology. 2007;132:294–300.
40. Migita K, Abiru S, Maeda Y, et al. Serum levels of interleukin-6 and its soluble receptors in patients with hepatitis C virus infection. Hum Immunol. 2006;67:27–32.
41. Fisher-Wellman KH, Neufer PD. Linking mitochondrial bioenergetics to insulin resistance via redox biology. Trends Endocrinol Metab. 2012;23:142–53.
42. Williams JA, Ding WX. A mechanistic review of mitophagy and its role in protection against alcoholic liver disease. Biomol Ther. 2015;5:2619–42.
43. Abdelmegeed MA, Ha SK, Choi Y, Akbar M, Song BJ. Role of CYP2E1 in mitochondrial dysfunction and hepatic tissue injury in alcoholic and non-alcoholic diseases. Curr Mol Pharmacol. 2017;10:207–25.
44. Donnelly KL, Smith CI, Schwarzenberg SJ, Jessurun J, Boldt MD, Parks EJ. Sources of fatty acids stored in liver and secreted vis lipoproteins in patients with nonalcoholic fatty liver disease. J Clin Invest. 2005;115:1343–51.
45. Lambert JE. Increased *de novo* lipogenesis is a distinct characteristic of individuals with nonalcoholic fatty liver disease. Gastroenterology. 2014;146:726–35.
46. Peterson RE, Kalavalapalli S, Williams CM, et al. Lipotoxicity in steatohepatitis occurs despite an increase in tricarboxylic acid cycle activity. Am J Physiol Endocrinol Metab. 2016;310:E484–94.

47. Satapati S, Sunny NE, Kucejova E, et al. Elevated TCA cycle function in the pathology of diet-induced hepatic insulin resitance and fatty liver. J Lipid Res. 2012;53:1081–92.
48. Sunny NE, Bril F, Cusi K. Mitochondrial adaptation in nonalcoholic fatty liver disease: novel mechanisms and treatment strategies. Trends Endoclinol Metab. 2017;28:250–60.
49. Satapati S, Kucejova B, Duarte JA, et al. Mitochondrial metabolism mediates oxidative stress in inflammation in fatty liver. J Clin Invest. 2015;125:4447–62.
50. Schwer B, Ren S, Pietschmann T, et al. Targeting of hepatitis C virus core protein to mitochondria through a novel C-terminal localization motif. J Virol. 2004;78:7958–68.
51. Korenaga M, Wang T, Li Y, et al. Hepatitis C virus core protein inhibits mitochondrial electron transport and increases reactive oxygen species (ROS) production. J Biol Chem. 2005;280:37481–8.
52. Tsutsumi T, Matsuda M, Aizaki H, et al. Proteomics analysis of mitochondrial proteins reveals overexpression of a mitochondrial protein chaperon, prohibitin, in cells expressing hepatitis C virus core protein. Hepatology. 2009;50:378–86.
53. Li Y, Boehning DF, Qian T, Popov VL, Weinman SA. Hepatitis C virus core protein increases mitochondrial ROS production by stimulation of Ca2+ uniporter activity. FASEB J. 2007;21:2474–85.
54. Piccoli C, Scrima R, Quarato G, et al. Hepatitis C virus protein expression causes calcium-mediated mitochondrial bioenergetic dysfunction and nitro-oxidative stress. Hepatology. 2007;46:58–65.
55. Pickles S, Vigie P, Youle R. Mitophagy and quality control mechanisms in mitochondrial maintenance. Curr Biol. 2018;28:R170–85.
56. Mizushima N, Levine B, Cuervo AM, Klionsky DJ. Autophagy fights disease through cellular self-digestion. Nature. 2008;451:1069–75.
57. Madrigal-Matute J, Cuevro AM. Regulation of liver metabolism by autophagy. Gastroenterology. 2016;150:328–39.
58. Maher P. Redox control of neural function: background, mechanisms, and significance. Antioxid Redox Signal. 2006;8:1941–70.
59. Sir D, Chen WL, Choi J, Wakita T, Yen TS, Ou JH. Induction of incomplete autophagic response by hepatitis C virus via the unfolded protein response. Hepatology. 2008;46:1054–61.
60. Hara Y, Yanatori I, Ikeda M, et al. Hepatitis C virus core protein suppresses mitophagy by interacting with Parkin in the context of mitochondrial depolarization. Am J Pathol. 2014;184:3026–39.

Chapter 11
Role of Apoptosis in Liver Diseases

Hayato Hikita and Tetsuo Takehara

Abstract In the livers of patients with various chronic hepatic diseases, including viral hepatitis, alcoholic liver disease and non-alcoholic fatty liver disease, hepatocyte apoptosis is frequently detected. Hepatocyte apoptosis is regulated by pro-apoptotic and anti-apoptotic bcl-2 family proteins. Among the anti-apoptotic proteins, Bcl-xL and Mcl-1 collaborate to prevent the activation of the mitochondrial apoptotic pathway and to maintain hepatocyte homeostasis. Hepatocyte apoptosis is directly linked with the progression of liver diseases, including liver fibrogenesis and liver tumorigenesis. The regulation of hepatocyte apoptosis is one of the therapeutic strategies to prevent the progression of chronic liver diseases. In in vitro and in vivo mouse models of non-alcoholic fatty liver disease, hepatocyte autophagy is suppressed by Rubicon overexpression leading to an increase in ER stress and hepatocyte apoptosis. Rubicon inhibition ameliorates the increase in ER stress and hepatocyte apoptosis. Rubicon overexpression is also observed in the livers of patients with non-alcoholic fatty liver disease. Rubicon-targeted improvement of hepatocyte autophagy may thus be a new therapeutic strategy for patients with non-alcoholic fatty liver disease. Therefore, further mechanistic insights into how hepatocyte apoptosis is executed in patients with different chronic liver diseases may lead to the discovery of new therapeutic strategies that can suppress the progression of chronic liver diseases.

Keywords Bcl-2 family proteins · Bcl-xL · Mcl-1 · Chronic hepatitis · Oxidative stress · Liver tumorigenesis · Rubicon · Autophagy · Non-alcoholic fatty liver disease · Non-alcoholic steatohepatitis

---

H. Hikita · T. Takehara (✉)
Osaka University, Graduate School of Medicine, Suita, Osaka, Japan
e-mail: hikita@gh.med.osaka-u.ac.jp; takehara@gh.med.osaka-u.ac.jp

H. Yoshiji, K. Kaji (eds.), *Alcoholic/Non-Alcoholic Digestive Diseases*,
https://doi.org/10.1007/978-981-13-1465-0_11

11.1 Induction of Hepatocyte Apoptosis

Apoptosis is known as active cell death because it is executed by cells in an ATP-dependent manner. The mitochondrion is an essential player in the execution of hepatocyte apoptosis and also serves as an important organelle for ATP production through oxygen consumption. All kinds of apoptotic stimuli are transmitted to the mitochondria by Bak/Bax activation. In other words, all apoptotic stimuli finally activate Bak/Bax, resulting in the formation of a pore on the outer membrane of the mitochondria, also known as mitochondrial outer membrane permeabilization (MOMP). Once the pore is formed by Bak/Bax activation, cytochrome c is released from the mitochondrial intermembrane space to form the apoptosome with apaf-1. The apoptosome cleaves caspase-9 to activate it, and cleaved caspase-9 further cleaves caspase-3/7 to activate and execute apoptosis. After Bak/Bax forms the pore, apoptosis is automatically executed without any protein transcription [1]. This step towards apoptosis after Bak/Bax activation is a common pathway among all hepatocyte apoptotic stimuli. However, pathways leading up to Bak/Bax activation are dependent on apoptotic stimuli. These pathways are broadly divided into two types. One is the extrinsic pathway through death receptors, and the other is the intrinsic pathway. In hepatocytes, three death receptors exist, namely TNF-α receptor, Fas and TRAIL receptor. These receptors are activated by their corresponding ligands, namely TNF-α, Fas ligand and TRAIL, respectively. The activation of these death receptors leads to the cleavage and activation of caspase-8. Activated caspase-8 truncates Bid, a BH3-only protein, and truncated-Bid (t-Bid) activates Bak/Bax. In the intrinsic pathway, several BH3-only proteins, including Bim, Puma, Noxa, Bmf, Bad, Bik and Hrk, work as stress sensors. Intracellular stress, such as endoplasmic reticulum (ER) stress, oxidative stress or genotoxic stress, transcriptionally or post-transcriptionally activates some BH3-only proteins. For example, ER stress transcriptionally and via phosphorylation activates Bim. Genotoxic stress transcriptionally activates Puma. These activated BH3-only proteins then activate Bak/Bax [1] (Fig. 11.1).

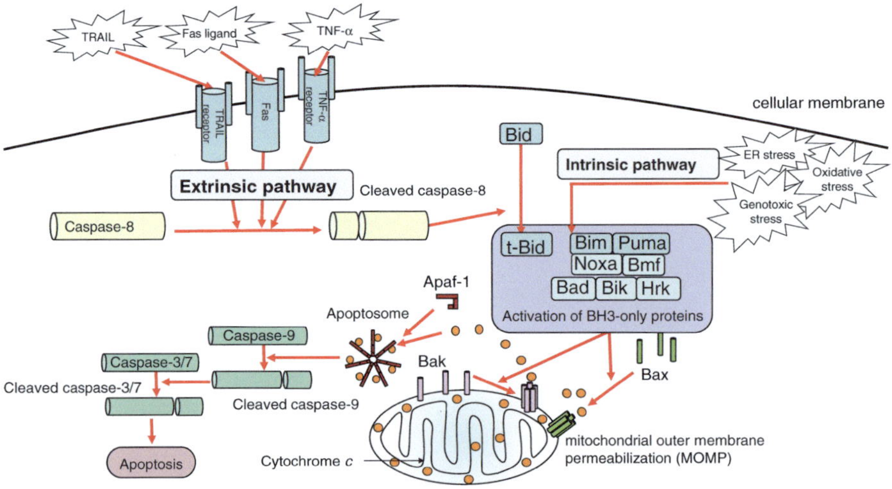

Fig. 11.1 Apoptosis signalling in hepatocytes

11.2 Anti-Apoptotic Bcl-2 Family Proteins for Apoptosis Inhibition

To suppress Bak/Bax activation, anti-apoptotic Bcl-2 family proteins exist in cells. Anti-apoptotic bcl-2 family proteins can bind both activated BH3-only proteins and Bak/Bax, and they directly or indirectly inhibit Bak/Bax activation. In mammalian cells, 5 anti-apoptotic Bcl-2 family proteins have been identified, namely Bcl-xL, Mcl-1, Bcl-2, Bfl-1 and Bcl-w. Mice with Bcl-2 [2], Bfl-1 [3] and Bcl-w [4, 5] knocked out have been generated but have not been reported to exhibit any phenotype in their livers, suggesting that these proteins do not have much of an effect on apoptosis in hepatocytes. In contrast, our previous study has clarified the importance of the anti-apoptotic bcl-2 family proteins Bcl-xL and Mcl-1 in hepatocyte apoptosis [6]. First, to examine the impact of Bcl-xL and Mcl-1 on hepatocytes, we generated hepatocyte-specific Bcl-xL or Mcl-1 knockout mice. Although hepatocyte-specific Bcl-xL or Mcl-1 hetero-deficient mice did not show any phenotype, hepatocyte-specific Bcl-xL or Mcl-1 homo-deficient mice displayed persistent hepatocyte apoptosis. TUNEL-positive hepatocytes were abundant in those murine livers [6, 7]. Additionally, the levels of cleaved caspase-3 as well as serum alanine aminotransferase (ALT) were increased in the hepatocyte-specific Bcl-xL or Mcl-1 homo-deficient mice. However, these phenotypes were completely abolished by further knockout of Bak/Bax. Interestingly, the deficiency of BH3-only proteins Bid or Bim also decreased hepatocyte apoptosis in Bcl-xL or Mcl-1 knockout mice [8, 9]. These results suggest that a small proportion of Bid and Bim are activated and that these proteins actively participate in hepatocyte apoptosis even under physiological settings. These data further show that the anti-apoptotic proteins Bcl-xL and Mcl-1 are important for maintaining hepatocyte homeostasis (Fig. 11.2). Bid is activated by death receptors. Since the liver is directly connected to the gut, many lipopolysaccharide (LPS) may be present in the portal vein. LPS constitutively activates death receptor in hepatocytes though Kupffer cell activation. This may be one reason why Bid is constitutively activated in hepatocytes. In addition, hepatocytes produce various proteins, which in turn increase ER stress. This may be another reason why Bim is constitutively activated in hepatocytes.

Next, to examine the interaction between Mcl-1 and Bcl-xL, we generated hepatocyte-specific Bcl-xL and Mcl-1 knockout mice. Although hepatocyte-specific Bcl-xL or Mcl-1 hetero-deficient mice did not show any phenotype as described above, hepatocyte-specific Bcl-xL and Mcl-1 double hetero-deficient mice displayed persistent hepatocyte apoptosis. Hepatocyte-specific Bcl-xL hetero-deficient and Mcl-1 homo-deficient mice, hepatocyte-specific Bcl-xL homo-deficient and Mcl-1 hetero-deficient mice or hepatocyte-specific Bcl-xL and Mcl-1 homo-deficient mice developed liver impairment, where most of the hepatocytes nearly disappeared at birth, and all these mice died within 1 day after birth [6]. Drug-inducible hepatocyte-specific Bcl-xL and Mcl-1 double knockout in mice causes severe acute hepatitis, where almost all hepatocytes undergo apoptosis, leading to death. In summary, deficiency of one allele among the total 4 alleles of Bcl-xL and Mcl-1 is not phenotypic, deficiency of two alleles results in constitutive hepatocyte apoptosis, and deficiency of more than two alleles causes liver impairment possibly

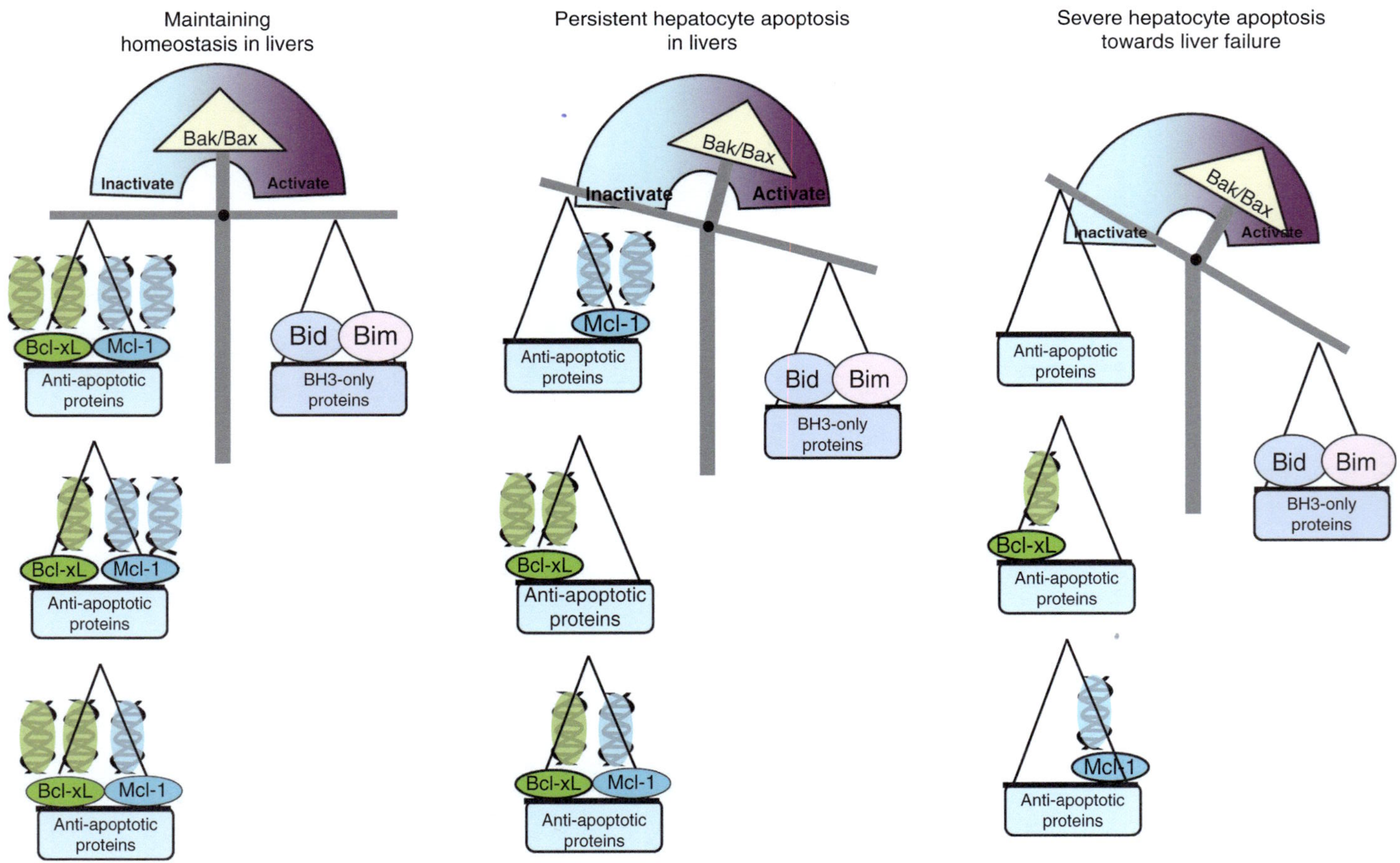

Fig. 11.2 The impact of Bcl-xL and Mcl-1 on hepatocyte homeostasis

by severe apoptosis. These results suggest that Bcl-xL and Mcl-1 are essential for hepatocytes and collaborate to protect hepatocytes from apoptosis (Fig. 11.2).

11.3 Impact of Persistent Hepatocyte Apoptosis in Liver Disease

In the livers of individuals with several chronic liver diseases, including chronic hepatitis C, chronic hepatitis B, alcoholic liver disease and non-alcoholic fatty liver disease (NAFLD), hepatocyte apoptosis is frequently detected. However, the impact of pure hepatocyte apoptosis is difficult to examine. To this end, the hepatocyte-specific Bcl-xL- and Mcl-1-deficient mice generated by us are useful since these mice display persistent hepatocyte apoptosis without any infection or stimulus. These mice demonstrate fibrotic change in their livers. These fibrotic changes can be attenuated via the inhibition of hepatocyte apoptosis by genetic ablation of a pro-apoptotic protein, such as Bak, Bax and Bid [1, 6, 8, 10, 11]. Surprisingly, these mice develop liver tumours after 1 year of age. Moreover, the tumourous lesions are similar to those of well-differentiated or moderately differentiated hepatocellular carcinoma in humans. Inhibition of hepatocyte apoptosis using genetic ablation of pro-apoptotic proteins, such as Bak, Bax and Bid, can also suppress liver tumourigenesis, indicating that persistent hepatocyte apoptosis is directly linked with the development of liver tumour [11, 12]. During the activation of hepatocyte apoptosis, not only caspase activity but also reactive oxygen species are increased, leading to an increase in oxidative stress in cells [11]. Persistent hepatocyte apoptosis increases oxidative stress in livers. The administration of anti-oxidants does not decrease hepatocyte apoptosis or fibrosis but significantly decreases liver tumourigenesis rates [11]. These results indicate that hepatocyte apoptosis is a sufficient factor for liver fibrosis and carcinogenesis and that hepatocyte apoptosis is not a bystander in progression of liver disease. Regulations of hepatocyte apoptosis is thus a useful strategy for treatment of chronic liver diseases.

11.4 Hepatocyte Apoptosis in Non-alcoholic Fatty Liver Diseases

In the livers of patients with NAFLD or non-alcoholic steatohepatitis (NASH), TUNEL-positive cells are detected [13]. The increase in TUNEL-positive hepatocytes is correlated with NASH severity [13]. In clinical trials, a caspase inhibitor decreases serum ALT levels in a dose-dependent manner in patients with NASH [14]. These data suggest that hepatocyte apoptosis is one of the characteristic features of NAFLD/NASH. In patients with NAFLD/NASH, several factors induce apoptosis. Free fatty acids induce ER stress and oxidative stress in hepatocytes leading to hepatocyte apoptosis through the intrinsic pathway [15]. This lipid overload-induced hepatocyte apoptosis is called lipoapoptosis. In patients with NAFLD/NASH, LPS levels in portal vein are increased [15], which results in an increase in cytokines and chemokines through toll-like receptor 4 on Kupffer cells. Among cytokines, TNF-α induces hepatocyte apoptosis through death receptor signalling [16]. Cytokines and chemokines also induce T or natural killer (NK) cell activation, which also stimulate hepatocyte death receptor signalling towards hepatocyte apoptosis [16]. Apoptotic hepatocytes release many kinds of extracellular vesicles as well as apoptotic bodies, both of which can directly or indirectly induce apoptosis in other hepatocytes [17]. Thus, many factors collaborate to induce hepatocyte apoptosis in patients with NAFLD/NASH.

11.5 Effect of Autophagy on Lipoapoptosis

Autophagy is a process by which proteins or organelles are degraded, and this process contributes to the maintenance of cellular homeostasis. We recently clarified the interaction between lipoapoptosis and autophagy and its underlying mechanism [18]. In that study, hepatocytes cultured with palmitic acid, a saturated free fatty acid, underwent lipoapoptosis with an increase in ER stress. This process also inhibited autophagy at the autophagosome and lysosome fusion step. To examine the underlying mechanisms by which palmitic acid impaired autophagy, we analysed autophagy-related proteins. The expression levels of Atg5 and Atg7, essential proteins for autophagy, were not changed by palmitic acids. The mTOR pathway, which negatively regulates autophagy, is inhibited by palmitic acids. The expression of Rubicon, another negative regulator of autophagy that inhibits the autophagosome and lysosome fusion step [19, 20], is increased by palmitic acid. Although the mRNA levels of Rubicon are not altered, the speed of degradation of Rubicon is decreased by palmitic acid. siRNA-mediated knockdown of Rubicon efficiently suppresses palmitic acid-induced Rubicon increase and autophagy impairment, as well as decreases palmitic acid-induced lipoapoptosis by reducing ER stress. These in vitro data suggest that palmitic acid increases Rubicon expression, leading to autophagy impairment, which contribute to an increase in ER stress and lipoapoptosis induction. Autophagy has also been reported to be involved in lipid metabolism by a process called lipophagy [21]. In our study, palmitic acid increased lipid droplet accumulation in hepatocytes, and this palmitic acid-induced lipid accumulation in hepatocytes was suppressed by siRNA-mediated Rubicon knockdown. These results may reflect impairments in lipophagy.

To examine the interaction between autophagy and lipoapoptosis in vivo, mice were given high-fat diet for 1–4 months. From 1 month onward after high-fat diet feeding, hepatocyte apoptosis increased with ER stress in mouse livers in a time-dependent manner. Additionally, in response to high-fat diet, the expression levels of p62 increased post-transcriptionally, and the number of autophagosomes also increased, suggesting that autophagy was impaired by high-fat diet feeding. Consistent with the in vitro data, high-fat diet did not affect atg5 and atg7 expression levels but inhibited the mTOR pathway and increased Rubicon expression levels without altering Rubicon mRNA levels in the liver. Although mice with hepatocyte-specific Rubicon knockout did not display any phenotypic changes regarding growth or liver histological features under physiological conditions, the increase in p62 expression levels in the livers was suppressed in response to high-fat diet, suggesting that high-fat diet-induced autophagy impairment can be suppressed by Rubicon knockout in hepatocytes. Hepatocyte-specific Rubicon deficiency suppressed lipoapoptosis and ER stress in mouse livers 4 months after high-fat diet feeding. Interestingly, compared with wild-type mice, hepatocyte-specific Rubicon knockout mice displayed a reduction in liver size and weight and decreased lipid droplet accumulation or triglyceride levels in hepatocytes in response to high-fat diet. However, compared with wild-type mice, hepatocyte-specific Rubicon knockout mice demonstrated an increase in gonadal fat pad weight. Based on these weight changes in the liver and fat tissues, rapid lipid metabolism by autophagy progression might result in the shuttling of lipids from hepatocytes to adipocytes. Further detailed analysis is needed regarding these processes.

Finally, we used clinical samples to further elucidate the underlying mechanisms. The expression of Rubicon and p62 was higher in the livers of patients with NAFLD than in the livers of patients without NAFLD, suggesting that the increase in Rubicon levels is also observed in humans and that this increase may contribute to NAFLD progression. Collectively, high-fat diet post-transcriptionally increases Rubicon expression, leading to autophagy impairment in hepatocytes, which increases both lipoapoptosis and lipid accumulation in hepatocytes (Fig. 11.3).

11.6 Conclusion

In the early days, apoptosis was considered a process of silent cell death, while necrosis, another type of cell death, was thought to spread many kinds of danger-associated molecular patterns (DAMPs) and induce severe inflammation. However, pure hepatocyte apoptosis is enough for the progression of liver disease towards fibrosis and carcinogenesis. Hepatocyte apoptosis is never a form of silent cell death. Thus, further mechanistic insights into how hepatocyte apoptosis is executed in patients with different chronic liver diseases may lead to the discovery of new therapeutic strategies that can suppress the progression of chronic liver diseases.

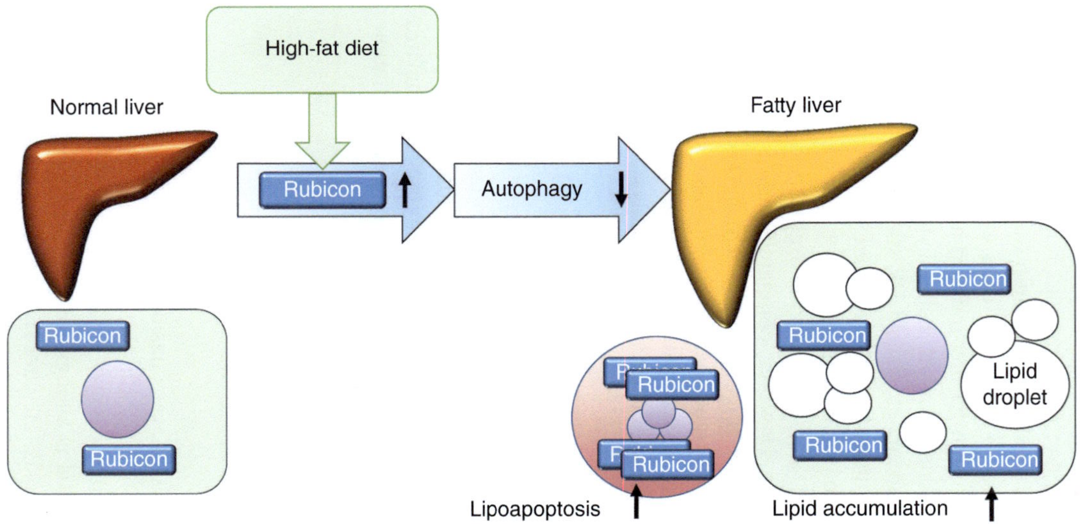

Fig. 11.3 High-fat diet increases Rubicon expression in hepatocytes, leading to autophagy impairment, which contributes to lipoapoptosis and lipid accumulation in hepatocytes

References

1. Hikita H, Takehara T. Regulation of apoptosis by bcl-2 family proteins in liver injury. In: Ding WX, Yin XM, editors. Molecules, systems and signaling in liver injury. Berlin: Springer; 2017. p. 53–74.
2. Veis DJ, Sorenson CM, Shutter JR, et al. Bcl-2-deficient mice demonstrate fulminant lymphoid apoptosis, polycystic kidneys, and hypopigmented hair. Cell. 1993;75:229–40.
3. Hamasaki A, Sendo F, Nakayama K, et al. Accelerated neutrophil apoptosis in mice lacking A1-a, a subtype of the bcl-2-related A1 gene. J Exp Med. 1998;188:1985–92.
4. Ross AJ, Waymire KG, Moss JE, et al. Testicular degeneration in bclw-deficient mice. Nat Genet. 1998;18:251–6.
5. Print CG, Loveland KL, Gibson L, et al. Apoptosis regulator bcl-w is essential for spermatogenesis but appears otherwise redundant. Proc Natl Acad Sci U S A. 1998;95:12424–31.
6. Hikita H, Takehara T, Shimizu S, et al. Mcl-1 and Bcl-xL cooperatively maintain integrity of hepatocytes in developing and adult murine liver. Hepatology. 2009;50:1217–26.
7. Takehara T, Tatsumi T, Suzuki T, et al. Hepatocyte-specific disruption of Bcl-xL leads to continuous hepatocyte apoptosis and liver fibrotic responses. Gastroenterology. 2004;127:1189–97.
8. Hikita H, Takehara T, Kodama T, et al. BH3-only protein bid participates in the Bcl-2 network in healthy liver cells. Hepatology. 2009;50:1972–80.
9. Kodama T, Hikita H, Kawaguchi T, et al. The Bcl-2 homology 3 (BH3)-only proteins Bim and Bid are functionally active and restrained by anti-apoptotic B-cell CLL/lymphoma 2 (Bcl-2) family proteins in healthy liver. J Biol Chem. 2013;288(42):30009–18.
10. Takehara T, Takahashi H. Suppression of Bcl-xL deamidation in human hepatocellular carcinomas. Cancer Res. 2003;63:3054–7.
11. Hikita H, Kodama T, Tanaka S, et al. Activation of the mitochondrial apoptotic pathway produces reactive oxygen species and oxidative damage in hepatocytes that contribute to liver tumorigenesis. Cancer Prev Res (Phila). 2015;8:693–701.
12. Hikita H, Kodama T, Shimizu S, et al. Bak deficiency inhibits liver carcinogenesis: a causal link between apoptosis and carcinogenesis. J Hepatol. 2012;57:92–100.
13. Feldstein AE, Canbay A, Angulo P, et al. Hepatocyte apoptosis and fas expression are prominent features of human nonalcoholic steatohepatitis. Gastroenterology. 2003;125:437–43.
14. Ratziu V, Sheikh MY, Sanyal AJ, et al. A phase 2, randomized, double-blind, placebo-controlled study of GS-9450 in subjects with nonalcoholic steatohepatitis. Hepatology. 2012;55:419–28.
15. Marra F, Svegliati-Baroni G. Lipotoxicity and the gut-liver axis in NASH pathogenesis. J Hepatol. 2018;68:280–95.
16. Win S, Than TA, Zhang J, et al. New insights into the role and mechanism of c-Jun-N-terminal kinase signaling in the pathobiology of liver diseases. Hepatology. 2017;67(5):2013–24.
17. Povero D, Feldstein AE. Novel molecular mechanisms in the development of non-alcoholic steatohepatitis. Diabetes Metab J. 2016;40(1):11.
18. Tanaka S, Hikita H, Tatsumi T, et al. Rubicon inhibits autophagy and accelerates hepatocyte apoptosis and lipid accumulation in nonalcoholic fatty liver disease. Hepatology. 2016;64(6):1994–2014.
19. Matsunaga K, Saitoh T, Tabata K, et al. Two Beclin 1-binding proteins, Atg14L and Rubicon, reciprocally regulate autophagy at different stages. Nat Cell Biol. 2009;11:385–96.
20. Zhong Y, Wang QJ, Li X, et al. Distinct regulation of autophagic activity by Atg14L and Rubicon associated with Beclin 1-phosphatidylinositol-3-kinase complex. Nat Cell Biol. 2009;11:468–76.
21. Singh R, Kaushik S, Wang Y, et al. Autophagy regulates lipid metabolism. Nature. 2009;458:1131–5.

Part III
Alcoholic/Non-Alcoholic Pancreatic Diseases

Chapter 12
Genetics of Pancreatitis

Atsushi Masamune and Tooru Shimosegawa

Abstract The association between alcohol misuse and chronic pancreatitis (CP) has been recognized for a long time. CP is a multifactorial and a complex disease, and the combination of genetic, environmental, and metabolic factors contributes to its development. Extensive research has been done to clarify the genetic factors. Candidate-gene approaches have focused on variants in the alcohol metabolizing enzymes (alcohol dehydrogenase 1B (*ADH1B*) and aldehyde dehydrogenase 2 (*ALDH2*)) and known pancreatitis susceptibility genes such as cationic trypsinogen (*PRSS1*), serine protease inhibitor Kazal type 1 (*SPINK1*), and chymotrypsin C (*CTRC*). It has been increasingly acknowledged that these previously known pancreatitis susceptibility genes identified in non-alcoholic (hereditary and idiopathic) CP also play a role in alcoholic CP. In addition, recent genome-wide association studies have identified new risk loci: the polymorphisms in the *PRSS1-PRSS2* and the *CLDN2-RIPPLY1-MORC4* loci and the inversion in the *CTRB1-CTRB2* locus. The genetic alterations might at least in part explain a long-standing unsolved question: why only a small portion of heavy drinkers develop pancreatitis.

Keywords Alcohol dehydrogenase · Aldehyde dehydrogenase · CTRB · CTRC
Genome-wide association study · Pancreatitis · PRSS1 · PRSS2 · SPINK1
Trypsin

The association between alcohol misuse and chronic pancreatitis (CP) has been recognized for a long time. Historically, alcohol misuse is the leading cause of CP and accounts for approximately 60–90% of the cases in industrialized nations worldwide [1]. However, only 1–5% of heavy drinkers develop pancreatitis, indicating that alcoholic pancreatitis is not caused by chronic alcohol misuse alone [2]. Some individuals may develop alcoholic pancreatitis with alcohol intake as low as 20 g/day, whereas most individuals do not develop pancreatitis no matter how long or how much they drink. CP is a multifactorial and a complex disease, and the

A. Masamune (✉) · T. Shimosegawa
Division of Gastroenterology, Tohoku University Graduate School of Medicine, Sendai, Japan
e-mail: amasamune@med.tohoku.ac.jp

H. Yoshiji, K. Kaji (eds.), *Alcoholic/Non-Alcoholic Digestive Diseases*,
https://doi.org/10.1007/978-981-13-1465-0_12

combination of genetic, environmental, and metabolic factors contribute to its development. Extensive research has been done to clarify the genetic factors [3, 4]. In addition to candidate-gene approaches focusing on variants in the alcohol metabolizing enzymes and known pancreatitis susceptibility genes such as *PRSS1*, *SPINK1*, and *CTRC*, genome-wide association studies (GWAS) have identified a new risk locus susceptible to CP. In this chapter, we review the genetics of pancreatitis, focusing on alcoholic CP.

12.1 Alcohol-Metabolizing Enzymes

Ethanol is oxidized to acetaldehyde by alcohol dehydrogenase (ADH), and acetaldehyde is further metabolized to acetate by aldehyde dehydrogenase (ALDH) [5]. These oxidization processes largely depend on ADH1B and ALDH2, respectively. ADH1B and ALDH2 are also expressed in pancreatic acinar cells [5]. In East Asian populations, the enzymatic activities of ADH1B and ALDH2 are regulated by the dysfunctional variants, rs1229984 (c.143A>G; p.H48R) and rs671 (c.1510G>A; p.E504K), respectively [6]. The reference allele *ADH1B*1* carries the amino acid arginine [Arg] and the *ADH1B*2* allele carries histidine [His] at the amino acid position 48. The *ADH1B*2* allele is very common in East Asian populations but rare in European populations. The *ADH2*1/*1* genotype encodes a less active form of ADH1B and the *ADH1B*2* allele encodes super-active forms of ADH1B. A meta-analysis showed that the *ADH1B*2* allele protects against alcohol dependence (Odds ratio = 0.44; $P < 10^{-36}$) and its frequency is lower in such patients in Asia [7]. In the case of the *ALDH2* gene, the reference allele *ALDH2*1* carries the amino acid glutamine [Glu] and the *ADH1B*2* allele carries lysine [Lys] at the amino acid positions 504 of the precursor protein (487 of the mature protein). In the presence of the *ALDH2*2* allele, the enzymatic activity of ALDH2 is severely compromised resulting in acetaldehyde accumulation, which enters the systemic circulation and initiates the commonly observed facial flushing syndrome [5, 6]. A strong protective effect of the *ALDH2*2* allele against alcoholism and alcohol-induced medical diseases has been shown [7]. Due to the delayed oxidation in the presence of the *ALDH2*2*, these individuals have high blood acetaldehyde concentrations, which can cause adverse reactions sufficient to deter drinking.

The impact of these dysfunctional variants in alcoholic CP has been studied mainly in Japan [8–10]. Overall, the frequency of the *ADH1B*1* allele in Japanese patients with alcoholic CP was significantly higher compared with controls, but lower than that in alcoholism without pancreatitis (Table 12.1). The frequency of the *ADH1B*1* allele was 0.29–0.39 in patients with alcoholic CP, 0.44–0.52 in alcoholic without CP, and 0.25 in 1070 controls (https://ijgvd.megabank.tohoku.ac.jp/). A recent GWAS from Europe revealed that the *ADH1B* p.H48R variant represents an alcohol dependence variant and is not associated with CP [11]. The frequency of the *ALDH2*2* allele was significantly lower in patients with alcoholic CP and in alcoholic subjects compared with healthy controls [8–10]. The frequency of the

Table 12.1 *ADH1B* and *ALDH2* genotypes in patients with alcoholic CP and controls in Japan

ADH1B	First author (year)	Population	*n*	*1/*1 (%)	*1/*2 (%)	*2/*2 (%)	*1allele frequency	*2allele frequency	Reference
Alcoholic CP	Matsumoto (1996)	Japan	52	11 (21.2)	19 (36.5)	22 (42.3)	0.39	0.61	[8]
	Shimosegawa (2008)	Japan	78	8 (10.2)	29 (37.2)	41 (52.6)	0.29	0.71	[9]
	Yokoyama (2013)	Japan	80	12 (14)	36 (44)	32 (39)	0.38	0.62	[10]
Alcoholic without CP	Matsumoto M (1996)	Japan	244	84 (34.4)	86 (35.2)	74 (30.3)	0.52	0.48	[8]
	Yokoyama A (2013)	Japan	1712	479 (28.0)	554 (32.4)	679 (39.7)	0.44	0.56	[9]
Healthy controls	Shimosegawa T (2008)	Japan	461	33 (7.2)	160 (34.7)	268 (58.1)	0.25	0.76	[10]
	ToMMo[a]	Japan	1070	69 (6.4)	406 (37.9)	595 (55.6)	0.25	0.75	
ALDH2	First author (year)	Race	*n*	*1/*1 (%)	*1/*2 (%)	*2/*2 (%)	*1allele frequency	*2allele frequency	Reference
Alcoholic CP	Matsumoto M (1996)	Japan	52	48 (92.3)	4 (7.7)	0 (0)	0.96	0.04	[8]
	Shimosegawa T (2008)	Japan	86	82 (95.3)	4 (4.7)	0 (0)	0.98	0.02	[9]
	Yokoyama A (2013)	Japan	80	72 (90)	8 (9)	0 (0)	0.94	0.06	[10]
Alcoholic without CP	Matsumoto M (1996)	Japan	244	210 (86.1)	34 (13.9)	0 (0)	0.93	0.07	[8]
	Yokoyama A (2013)	Japan	1712	1442 (84.2)	270 (15.8)	0 (0)	0.92	0.08	[9]
Healthy controls	Shimosegawa T (2008)	Japan	461	268 (58.1)	162 (35.1)	31 (6.7)	0.76	0.24	[10]
	ToMMo[a]	Japan	1070	772 (72.1)	318 (29.7)	40 (3.7)	0.81	0.19	

[a]https://ijgvd.megabank.tohoku.ac.jp/

*ALDH2*2/*2* genotype was 0 in both patients with alcoholic CP and alcoholics without CP, whereas it was 0.037 in 1070 controls. Importantly, the low frequency of the *ALDH2*2* allele in patients with alcoholic CP might be associated with alcoholism, but not specifically with alcoholic CP. Indeed, Yokoyama et al. [10] reported that the frequencies of the *ADH1B*2* allele carriers and ALDH2*1/*1 carriers tended to be higher in alcoholic CP patients than in alcoholic patients without CP, but the differences were not statistically significant.

12.2 PRSS1

PRSS1 encodes cationic trypsinogen, the most abundant isoform of trypsinogen in human pancreatic juice. In 1996, Whitcomb et al. [12] identified the p.R122H (c.365G>A) mutation in the *PRSS1* gene as a cause of hereditary pancreatitis. The p.R122H mutation is the most common one, followed by the p.N29I (c.86A>T) mutation. In Japan, a patient having the *PRSS1* p.R122H or p.N29I mutation is diagnosed as having hereditary pancreatitis even in the absence of family history of pancreatitis [13].

In addition to these hereditary pancreatitis-causing mutations, rare *PRSS1* variants have been reported in pancreatitis patients [14]. Among them, the *PRSS1* p.G208A (c.623G>C) variant has been reported mainly from Asia. Endoplasmic reticulum stress in pancreatic acinar cells resulting from the misfolding of the mutated PRSS1 protein is thought to be the underlying mechanism for the increased risk of pancreatitis [14]. A report from Japan showed that the *PRSS1* p.G208A variant was overrepresented in patients with alcoholic CP as well as in those with non-alcoholic CP [15]. The *PRSS1* p.G208A variant was found in 9/198 (4.5%) patients with idiopathic CP and 8/232 (3.4%) patients with alcoholic CP, whereas it was found in 1/411 (0.2%) controls. To date, this is the only reported association between the *PRSS1* variants and alcoholic CP.

12.3 SPINK1

The serine protease inhibitor Kazal type 1 (SPINK1), also known as pancreatic secretory trypsin inhibitor, is an acute-phase protein that is expressed in pancreatic acinar cells. SPINK1 acts as the first line of defense against prematurely activated intracellular trypsinogen by inhibiting up to 20% of trypsin activity within the pancreas [16]. In 2000, Witt et al. [17] reported that the *SPINK1* p.N34S (c.101A>G) variants were overrepresented in patients with early-onset idiopathic CP. Thereafter, it has been established that the *SPINK1* p.N34S variant is associated with non-alcoholic CP including idiopathic, familial, and tropical CP [3, 18, 19]. In addition

Table 12.2 Allele frequency of the *SPINK1* p.N34S variant in patients with alcoholic CP and controls

First author (year)	Population	Cases	Controls	Odds ratio (95% CI)	*P* value	Reference
Witt (2001)	UK-Germany-Switzerland	16/548	4/1080	8.09 (2.69–24.32)	0.00	[20]
Threadgold (2002)	EUROPAC	4/134	5/400	2.43 (0.64–9.19)	0.19	[21]
Drenth (2002)	Nederland	5/144	2/240	4.28 (0.82–22.36)	0.08	[22]
Schneider (2003)	USA	2/64	5/380	2.42 (0.46–12.75)	0.30	[23]
Perri (2003)	Italy	1/90	0/68	2.30 (0.09–57.24)	0.61	[24]
Chandak (2004)	India	11/82	8/580	11.08 (4.31–28.46)	0.00	[25]
Lempinen (2005)	Finland	9/174	12/918	4.12 (1.71–9.93)	0.00	[26]
Kume (2005)	Japan	0/64	1/330	0.59 (0.02–14.58)	1.00	[27]

EUROPAC: European Registry of Hereditary Pancreatitis and Pancreatic Cancer.

to non-alcoholic CP, the association of the *SPINK1* p.N34S variant with alcoholic CP has been reported in some studies, although the overall association was shown to be smaller than that with non-alcoholic CP (Table 12.2) [19–27]. A meta-analysis showed that the risk of alcoholic CP is about five times higher in the presence of the *SPINK1* p.N34S variant [19]. The contribution of the *SPINK1* p.N34S variant to alcoholic CP [Odds ratio = 4.98 (95% confidence interval: 3.16–7.85)] was smaller than that in idiopathic CP [Odds ratio = 14.97 (95% confidence interval: 9.09–24.67)].

The second most common variant, c.194+2T>C (IVS3+2T>C) has been reported in patients with CP [27]. The high frequency of this variant in pancreatitis patients is a characteristic feature of the *SPINK1* variant in East Asia including Japan. A Japanese study showed that the *SPINK1* c.194+2T>C variant was overrepresented in patients with alcoholic CP; it was found in 4/129 (3.1%) patients with alcoholic CP, but in none of 540 controls [18]. It has been suggested that the pathogenic *SPINK1* variants might result in altered interaction between SPINK1 and trypsin, thus affecting the protease/antiprotease balance within the pancreas [17]. However, the underlying mechanism linking the *SPINK1* p.N34S variant and pancreatitis remains unknown. On the other hand, the c.194+2T>C variant, which affects the consensus splicing site, causes the skipping of exon 3, where the coding region for the trypsin-binding site is located [28]. It is reasonable to assume that the mutated SPINK1 loses its inhibitory activity on trypsin, because it cannot bind to trypsin.

12.4 PRSS2

PRSS2 is another major trypsinogen isoform constituting the bulk of secreted trypsinogen in humans [29]. CP and alcoholism lead to a characteristic reversal of the isoform ratio, and anionic trypsinogen becomes the predominant zymogen secreted [16]. In 2006, Witt et al. [30] reported that the *PRSS2* p.G191R (c.571G > A) variant was less frequent in patients with CP [32/2466 (1.3%)] than in controls [220/6459 (3.4%)] in Europe. Upon activation by enterokinase or trypsin, purified recombinant p.G191R protein showed a complete loss of trypsin activity owing to the introduction of a new tryptic cleavage site that renders the enzyme hypersensitive to autocatalytic proteolysis. Therefore, the *PRSS2* p.G191R variant leads to rapid trypsin autodegradation and protects against CP. This study was also replicated in Japanese patients with CP [31]. The frequency of the *PRSS2* p.G191R variant was 1/244 (0.4%) in patients with CP, while it was 26/402 (6.5%) in the control population. The differences were still significant even when the patients were stratified based on the etiology ($P = 0.009$ for alcoholic CP vs. Controls, and $P = 0.01$ for idiopathic CP vs. Controls). Thus, the *PRSS2* p.G191R variant may protect against CP in the Japanese population, as well.

12.5 CTRC

Chymotrypsin C (CTRC) is a minor isoform of chymotrypsin, which degrades all human trypsin and trypsinogen isoforms with high specificity [32]. CTRC serves as a second line of defense against premature activation of the trypsinogen isoform. Rosendahl et al. [32] reported that the p.R254W (c.760C>T) or the micro-deletion variant p.K247_R254del (c.738_761del24) in the *CTRC* gene was found in 3.3% of patients with idiopathic CP or HP, whereas they were found in only 0.7% of the controls. In a replication cohort, these two variants (p.R254W and p.K247_R254del) were found more frequently in patients with alcoholic CP (2.9%) than in subjects with alcohol-related liver disease (0.7%) ($P = 0.02$). Of note, there are geographical differences in the spectrum of the *CTRC* variants [32, 33]. In India, the p.A73T (c.217G>A) and the p.V251I (c.703G>A) variants were the most common ones. These common variants in Europe and India are very rare in Japanese subjects and only one out of the 506 CP patients had the p.R254W variant [33]. On the other hand, a novel missense variant p.R29Q (c.86G>A) was found in a patient with alcoholic CP. Functional analysis showed that the p.R29Q variant was catalytically inactive due to the loss of activation by trypsin [34]. These results support the notion that there is an imbalance of the protease/anti-protease system in alcoholic CP as well as in idiopathic CP.

LaRusch et al. [35] reported that the synonymous *CTRC* variant c.180C>T (p.G60=) was significantly overrepresented in CP of all etiologies, but not in recurrent acute pancreatitis as compared with controls (16.8% in CP, 11.9% in recurrent acute pancreatitis, 10.8% in controls). The *CTRC* c.180T allele was overrepresented in alcoholic CP patients (20.8%) compared to non-alcoholic CP patients (12.4%) [Odds ratio = 1.9 (95% confidence interval: 1.30–2.79)]. This finding suggests that the *CTRC* c.180 T variant acts as a disease modifier that promotes the progression from recurrent acute pancreatitis to CP in alcoholic patients.

12.6 CFTR

The cystic fibrosis transmembrane conductance regulator (*CFTR*) gene, responsible for the development of cystic fibrosis, is known as a pancreatitis susceptibility gene [36, 37]. Audrézet et al. [38] reported from France that at least 20% of the patients with idiopathic CP carried one of the most common *CFTR* mutations. However, genetic studies supporting the role of the *CFTR* variants in alcoholic CP are scarce. Along this line, it has been increasingly recognized that compound and trans-heterozygosity in the pancreatitis susceptibility genes are an overt risk factor for idiopathic CP [39]. From this point of view, the pathogenic roles of the *CFTR* variants might have been overestimated [39]. Although alcohol consumption has been shown to impair the CFTR function in pancreatic ductal cells and sensitize the organ to injury in mice and humans [40], the role of the CFTR variants in alcoholic CP in genetics requires further clarification.

12.7 GWAS

GWAS overcomes the limitations of a pathophysiology-based candidate gene approach, enabling the discovery of new and unsuspected pancreatitis susceptibility genes. In 2013, Whitcomb et al. [41] reported the first GWAS employing 676 CP patients and 4507 controls (first cohort), and 910 CP or recurrent acute pancreatitis patients and 4170 controls (second cohort). This study identified that the polymorphisms in the *PRSS1-PRSS2* locus (rs10273639) and the claudin 2 locus (*CLDN2-RIPPLY1-MORC4* locus rs7057398 and rs12688220) conferred an increased risk of alcoholic CP especially in men, but not of alcohol-associated cirrhosis or alcohol dependence. The *PRSS1-PRSS2* rs10273639 T allele appeared to protect against CP by altering the expression of the trypsinogen gene, whereas the *RIPPLY1* rs7057398 C allele and *MORC4* rs12688220 T allele increased disease susceptibility through the atypical localization of claudin-2 in pancreatic acinar cells. Because *CLDN2* genotypes in the homozygous state in women or hemizygous one in men confer the greatest risk, this association might, at least in part, explain the male-dominancy in alcoholic CP. The association of alcoholic CP with polymorphisms in these loci has been replicated in Europe, Japan, and India [42–44], indicating that they are susceptible factors in alcoholic CP worldwide. The *CLDN2-RIPPLY1-MORC4* high-risk allele locus indicates a protease-independent mechanism that can increase the risk of pancreatitis. Obviously, further studies are warranted to elucidate the underlying mechanism.

A subsequent GWAS from Europe showed a novel association between alcoholic CP and polymorphisms in the genes encoding fucosyltransferase 2 non-secretor status (*FUT2* locus rs632111 and rs601338) and blood group B (*ABO* locus rs8176693) [45]. In 2017, Rosendhal et al. [11] reported another GWAS of 1959 alcoholic CP patients in Europe. The study replicated the association of alcoholic CP with the previously known risk loci including *CLDN2-MORC4*, *CTRC*, *PRSS1-PRSS2*, and *SPINK1*. The association was essentially unchanged when alcoholic CP patients were separately compared with chronic alcoholics and non-alcoholic controls. In addition, they identified the inversion in the *CTRB1-CTRB2* (chymotrypsin B1 and B2) locus in alcoholic and non-alcoholic CP. The inversion changes the expression ratio of the CTRB1 and CTRB2 isoforms, and thereby affects the protective trypsinogen degradation and ultimately pancreatitis risk.

12.8 Conclusions

It has been increasingly acknowledged that the previously known pancreatitis susceptibility genes identified in non-alcoholic (hereditary and idiopathic) CP also play a role in alcoholic CP (Table 12.3). The genetic variants in these susceptibility

Table 12.3 Genetic susceptibility factors in alcoholic CP

Mutation/polymorphism	Approach	References
PRSS1		
p.G208A	Candidate gene	[15]
SPINK1		
p.N34S	Candidate gene	[19, 20]
c.194 + 2 T > C	Candidate gene	[18]
PRSS2		
p.G191R	Candidate gene	[30, 31]
CTRC		
p.R254W, p.K247_R254del	Candidate gene	[32]
c.180C > T (p.G60=)	Candidate gene	[35]
CLDN2-RIPPLY1-MORC4 locus		
rs7057398, rs12688220	GWAS (two-stage)	[41–44]
ABO locus		
rs8176693	GWAS (two-stage)	[45]
FUT2 locus		
rs632111	GWAS (two-stage)	[45]
rs601338	GWAS (two-stage)	[45]
CTRB1-CTRB2 locus		
	GWAS (two-stage)	[11]

genes, especially those highly expressed in the pancreas, might at least in part explain a long-standing unsolved question: why only a small portion of heavy drinkers develop pancreatitis [2]. Elucidation of the genetic factors based on the genome-wide or exosome-wide approach will contribute to the identification of unexpected pancreatitis susceptibility genes, the pathogenesis of pancreatitis, and eventually to the development of new therapeutic options for pancreatitis.

Conflict of Interest None declared.

References

1. Yadav D, Lowenfels AB. The epidemiology of pancreatitis and pancreatic cancer. Gastroenterology. 2013;144:1252–61.
2. Lankisch PG, Lowenfels AB, Maisonneuve P. What is the risk of alcoholic pancreatitis in heavy drinkers? Pancreas. 2002;25:411–2.
3. Whitcomb DC. Genetic risk factors for pancreatic disorders. Gastroenterology. 2013;144:1292–302.
4. Aghdassi AA, Weiss FU, Mayerle J, et al. Genetic susceptibility factors for alcohol-induced chronic pancreatitis. Pancreatology. 2015;15:S23–31.
5. Chiang CP, Wu CW, Lee SP, et al. Expression pattern, ethanol-metabolizing activities, and cellular localization of alcohol and aldehyde dehydrogenases in human pancreas: implications for pathogenesis of alcohol-induced pancreatic injury. Alcohol Clin Exp Res. 2009;33:1059–68.
6. Hurley TD, Edenberg HJ. Genes encoding enzymes involved in ethanol metabolism. Alcohol Res. 2012;34:339–44.
7. Li D, Zhao H, Gelernter J. Strong association of the alcohol dehydrogenase 1B gene (ADH1B) with alcohol dependence and alcohol-induced medical diseases. Biol Psychiatry. 2011;70:504–12.
8. Matsumoto M, Takahashi H, Maruyama K, et al. Genotypes of alcohol-metabolizing enzymes and the risk for alcoholic chronic pancreatitis in Japanese alcoholics. Alcohol Clin Exp Res. 1996;20:289A–92A.
9. Shimosegawa T, Kume K, Masamune A. SPINK1, ADH2, and ALDH2 gene variants and alcoholic chronic pancreatitis in Japan. J Gastroenterol Hepatol. 2008;23:S82–6.
10. Yokoyama A, Mizukami T, Matsui T, et al. Genetic polymorphisms of alcohol dehydrogenase-1B and aldehyde dehydrogenase-2 and liver cirrhosis, chronic calcific pancreatitis, diabetes mellitus, and hypertension among Japanese alcoholic men. Alcohol Clin Exp Res. 2013;37:1391–401.
11. Rosendahl J, Kirsten H, Hegyi E, et al. Genome-wide association study identifies inversion in the CTRB1-CTRB2 locus to modify risk for alcoholic and non-alcoholic chronic pancreatitis. Gut. 2017;67(10):1855–63.. pii: gutjnl-2017-314454.
12. Whitcomb DC, Gorry MC, Preston RA, et al. Hereditary pancreatitis is caused by a mutation in the cationic trypsinogen gene. Nat Genet. 1996;14:141–5.
13. Masamune A, Kikuta K, Hamada S, et al. Nationwide survey of hereditary pancreatitis in Japan. J Gastroenterol. 2018;53:152–60.
14. Schnúr A, Beer S, Witt H, et al. Functional effects of 13 rare PRSS1 variants presumed to cause chronic pancreatitis. Gut. 2014;63:337–43.
15. Masamune A, Nakano E, Kume K, et al. PRSS1 c.623G>C (p.G208A) variant is associated with pancreatitis in Japan. Gut. 2014;63:366.
16. Rinderknecht H. Activation of pancreatic zymogens. Normal activation, premature intrapancreatic activation, protective mechanisms against inappropriate activation. Dig Dis Sci. 1986;31:314–21.

17. Witt H, Luck W, Hennies HC, et al. Mutations in the gene encoding the serine protease inhibitor, Kazal type 1 are associated with chronic pancreatitis. Nat Genet. 2000;25:213–6.
18. Masamune A. Genetics of pancreatitis: the 2014 update. Tohoku J Exp Med. 2014;232:69–77.
19. Aoun E, Chang CC, Greer JB, et al. Pathways to injury in chronic pancreatitis: decoding the role of the high-risk SPINK1 N34S haplotype using meta-analysis. PLoS One. 2008;3:e2003.
20. Witt H, Luck W, Becker M, et al. Mutation in the SPINK1 trypsin inhibitor gene, alcohol use, and chronic pancreatitis. JAMA. 2001;285:2716–7.
21. Threadgold J, Greenhalf W, Ellis I, et al. The N34S mutation of SPINK1 (PSTI) is associated with a familial pattern of idiopathic chronic pancreatitis but does not cause the disease. Gut. 2002;50:675–81.
22. Drenth JP, te Morsche R, Jansen JB. Mutations in serine protease inhibitor Kazal type 1 are strongly associated with chronic pancreatitis. Gut. 2002;50:687–92.
23. Schneider A, Pfützer RH, Barmada MM, et al. Limited contribution of the SPINK1 N34S mutation to the risk and severity of alcoholic chronic pancreatitis: a report from the United States. Dig Dis Sci. 2003;48:1110–5.
24. Perri F, Piepoli A, Stanziale P, et al. Mutation analysis of the cystic fibrosis transmembrane conductance regulator (CFTR) gene, the cationic trypsinogen (PRSS1) gene, and the serine protease inhibitor, Kazal type 1 (SPINK1) gene in patients with alcoholic chronic pancreatitis. Eur J Hum Genet. 2003;11:687–92.
25. Chandak GR, Idris MM, Reddy DN, et al. Absence of PRSS1 mutations and association of SPINK1 trypsin inhibitor mutations in hereditary and non-hereditary chronic pancreatitis. Gut. 2004;53:723–8.
26. Lempinen M, Paju A, Kemppainen E, et al. Mutations N34S and P55S of the SPINK1 gene in patients with chronic pancreatitis or pancreatic cancer and in healthy subjects: a report from Finland. Scand J Gastroenterol. 2005;40:225–30.
27. Kume K, Masamune A, Mizutamari H, et al. Mutations in the serine protease inhibitor Kazal Type 1 (SPINK1) gene in Japanese patients with pancreatitis. Pancreatology. 2005;5:354–60.
28. Kume K, Masamune A, Kikuta K, et al. [−215G>A; IVS3+2T>C] mutation in the SPINK1 gene causes exon 3 skipping and loss of the trypsin binding site. Gut. 2006;55:1214.
29. Kukor Z, Tóth M, Sahin-Tóth M. Human anionic trypsinogen: properties of autocatalytic activation and degradation and implications in pancreatic diseases. Eur J Biochem. 2003;270:2047–58.
30. Witt H, Sahin-Tóth M, Landt O, et al. A degradation-sensitive anionic trypsinogen (PRSS2) variant protects against chronic pancreatitis. Nat Genet. 2006;38:668–73.
31. Kume K, Masamune A, Takagi Y, et al. A loss-of-function p.G191R variant in the anionic trypsinogen (PRSS2) gene in Japanese patients with pancreatic disorders. Gut. 2009;58:820–4.
32. Rosendahl J, Witt H, Szmola R, et al. Chymotrypsin C (CTRC) variants that diminish activity or secretion are associated with chronic pancreatitis. Nat Genet. 2008;40:78–82.
33. Masamune A, Nakano E, Kume K, et al. Identification of novel missense CTRC variants in Japanese patients with chronic pancreatitis. Gut. 2013;62:653–4.
34. Szabó A, Ludwig M, Hegyi E, et al. Mesotrypsin signature mutation in a chymotrypsin C (CTRC) variant associated with chronic pancreatitis. J Biol Chem. 2015;290:17282–92.
35. LaRusch J, Lozano-Leon A, Stello K, et al. The common chymotrypsinogen C (CTRC) variant G60G (C.180T) increases risk of chronic pancreatitis but not recurrent acute pancreatitis in a north American population. Clin Transl Gastroenterol. 2015;6:e68.
36. Sharer N, Schwarz M, Malone G, et al. Mutations of the cystic fibrosis gene in patients with chronic pancreatitis. N Engl J Med. 1998;339:645–52.
37. Cohn JA, Friedman KJ, Noone PG, Knowles MR, Silverman LM, Jowell PS. Relation between mutations of the cystic fibrosis gene and idiopathic pancreatitis. N Engl J Med. 1998;339:653–8.
38. Audrézet MP, Chen JM, Le Maréchal C, et al. Determination of the relative contribution of three genes-the cystic fibrosis transmembrane conductance regulator gene, the cationic tryp-

sinogen gene, and the pancreatic secretory trypsin inhibitor gene-to the etiology of idiopathic chronic pancreatitis. Eur J Hum Genet. 2002;10:100–6.
39. Rosendahl J, Landt O, Bernadova J, et al. CFTR, SPINK1, CTRC and PRSS1 variants in chronic pancreatitis: is the role of mutated CFTR overestimated? Gut. 2013;62:582–92.
40. Maléth J, Balázs A, Pallagi P, et al. Alcohol disrupts levels and function of the cystic fibrosis transmembrane conductance regulator to promote development of pancreatitis. Gastroenterology. 2015;148:427–39.e16.
41. Whitcomb DC, LaRusch J, Krasinskas AM, et al. Common genetic variants in the CLDN2 and PRSS1-PRSS2 loci alter risk for alcohol-related and sporadic pancreatitis. Nat Genet. 2012;44:1349–54.
42. Derikx MH, Kovacs P, Scholz M, et al. Polymorphisms at PRSS1-PRSS2 and CLDN2-MORC4 loci associate with alcoholic and non-alcoholic chronic pancreatitis in a European replication study. Gut. 2015;64:1426–33.
43. Masamune A, Nakano E, Hamada S, et al. Common variants at PRSS1-PRSS2 and CLDN2-MORC4 loci associate with chronic pancreatitis in Japan. Gut. 2015;64:1345–6.
44. Giri AK, Midha S, Banerjee P, et al. Common variants in CLDN2 and MORC4 genes confer disease susceptibility in patients with chronicpancreatitis. PLoS One. 2016;11:e0147345.
45. Weiss FU, Schurmann C, Guenther A, et al. Fucosyltransferase 2 (FUT2) non-secretor status and blood group B are associated with elevated serum lipase activity in asymptomatic subjects, and an increased risk for chronic pancreatitis: a genetic association study. Gut. 2015;64:646–56.

Chapter 13
New Perspective in Pancreatic Cancer

Kota Nakamura, Takahiro Akahori, Minako Nagai, Satoshi Nishiwada, Kenji Nakagawa, Naoya Ikeda, and Masayuki Sho

Abstract Pancreatic cancer is a major cause of cancer-associated mortality. In recent years, improvement of chemotherapy provided better prognosis for the patient with both resectable and unresectable pancreatic cancer. This review discusses new perspective in all aspects of treatment for pancreatic cancer.

Keyword Pancreatic cancer · Treatment · Systemic chemotherapy · Surgery Adjuvant chemotherapy

13.1 Introduction

Pancreatic cancer, also known as pancreatic ductal adenocarcinoma, is the most common malignancy of the pancreas. In 2015, an estimate of 367,000 new cases were diagnosed worldwide and 359,000 people died from pancreatic cancer [1]. Pancreatic cancer is likely to become the second leading cause of cancer-related death by 2030, in the United States [2]. At diagnosis, 40–60% of patients present with metastatic disease, 30–40% present with borderline resectable pancreatic cancer (BRPC) and locally advanced pancreatic cancer (LAPC), and only 20–30% present with localized, potentially curable, and resectable tumors [1].

As surgery remains only potentially curative option for pancreatic cancer, the identification of BRPC as a clinical boundary may be essential to clarify a distinction along the continuum between technically resectable and locally advanced unresectable cancers. As clear definitions of BRPC and LAPC were lacking in the past, in 2014, the International Study Group for Pancreatic Surgery revised the definition of BRPC and LAPC [3], and these definitions were subsequently adopted by National Comprehensive Cancer Network [4, 5]. Categorizing the tumor resectability whether a margin-negative resection is possible to achieve with major vascular resection or truly unresectable from anatomic and biologic standpoints became a critical issue of the initial patient evaluation. While it is only in resectable pancreatic

K. Nakamura · T. Akahori · M. Nagai · S. Nishiwada · K. Nakagawa · N. Ikeda · M. Sho (✉)
Department of Surgery, Nara Medical University, Kashihara, Nara, Japan
e-mail: m-sho@naramed-u.ac.jp

H. Yoshiji, K. Kaji (eds.), *Alcoholic/Non-Alcoholic Digestive Diseases*,
https://doi.org/10.1007/978-981-13-1465-0_13

cancer that better prognosis was enjoyed by surgery, therapeutic managements of BRPC and LAPC were controversial despite significant advances in systemic chemotherapy in recent years. This review summarizes recent progress in the treatment of pancreatic cancer.

13.2 Chemotherapy for Metastatic or Locally Advanced Pancreatic Cancer

In 1997, gemcitabine became the standard treatment for advanced pancreatic cancer after a randomized trial showed significant improvement in the median overall survival (OS) as compared with fluorouracil administered as an intravenous bolus (5.6 vs. 4.4 months, $P = 0.002$) [6]. Since then, a number of phase III trials of newer cytotoxic or biologic agents combined with gemcitabine failed to show any survival improvement compared with gemcitabine alone. However, in 2007, the phase III trial of erlotinib plus gemcitabine versus gemcitabine alone demonstrated statistically significantly improved survival in advanced pancreatic cancer [7]. OS based on an intent-to-treat analysis was significantly prolonged on the erlotinib/gemcitabine arm with a hazard ratio (HR) of 0.82 (95% CI, 0.69–0.99; $P = 0.038$, median 6.2 vs 5.9 months). In 2011, the phase II-III trial of FOLFIRINOX versus gemcitabine alone showed a clinically meaningful improvement in survival [8]. The median OS was 11.1 months in the FOLFIRINOX group as compared with 6.8 months in the gemcitabine group ($P < 0.001$). Furthermore, a large-scale phase III study (GEST study) was conducted in patients with metastatic or locally advanced pancreatic cancer in Japan and Taiwan [9]. Although the non-inferiority of S-1 to GEM was confirmed (HR = 0.96; 97.5% CI, 0.78–0.18; $P < 0.001$), GS therapy did not demonstrate the superiority to GEM in OS (HR = 0.88; 97.5% CI, 0.71–1.08; $P = 0.15$). Based on the results of the GEST study, S-1 was accepted as an option in the treatment of metastatic or locally advanced pancreatic cancer in Japan. In addition, a phase III study showed that nab-paclitaxel plus gemcitabine significantly improved OS [10]. The median OS was 8.5 months in the nab-paclitaxel–gemcitabine group as compared with 6.7 months in the gemcitabine group (HR = 0.72; 95% CI, 0.62–0.83; $P < 0.001$) (Table 13.1).

Table 13.1 Systemic chemotherapy for metastatic pancreatic cancer

Year	Regimens	Outcome
1997	Gemcitabine vs fluorouracil	mOS 5.6 vs. 4.4 mo ($P = 0.002$)
2007	Erlotinib plus gemcitabine vs gemcitabine	mOS 6.2 vs 5.9 mo ($P = 0.038$)
2011	FOLFIRINOX versus gemcitabine	mOS 11.1 vs. 6.8 mo ($P < 0.001$)
2013	Nab-paclitaxel plus gemcitabine vs gemcitabine	mOS 8.5 vs. 6.7 mo ($P < 0.001$)

mOS median overall survival, *mo* months, *FOLFIRINOX* 5-fluorouracil, leucovorin, irinotecan, and oxaliplatin

13.3 Surgery

Despite significant improvement of chemotherapy provided better prognosis for the patient with pancreatic cancer during the past decade, surgery remains the only potentially curative treatment of localized diseases [11]. In early stage pancreatic cancer, the patients who were not offered surgery had worse survival than patients who underwent pancreatectomy [12]. For further survival benefits provided by surgery, various treatment strategies for localized pancreatic cancer are actively investigated.

13.3.1 *Extended Lymphadenectomy*

Regional pancreatectomy, first described by Fortner in 1973 in radical cancer surgery, had been developed in Japan [13] and Western countries [14–17]. Fortner's concept of regional pancreatectomy had a major impact on the clinical practice of pancreatic surgeons. Furthermore, the benefits of extended radical pancreatectomy have been evaluated and various results of retrospective studies have been reported. The prospective randomized controlled trial to compare the results of extended lymphadenectomy versus standard in radical pancreatoduodenectomy for pancreatic cancer was reported by Pedrazzoli [14], followed by Yeo and Farnell [15, 17]. Although many pancreatic surgeons had regarded extended pancreatectomy to be better than standard pancreatectomy, these randomized controlled studies demonstrated that extended pancreatectomy had no survival advantages compared with standard pancreatectomy. However, these randomized controlled trials had several limitations such as small numbers of patients and different extents of clearance of lymph nodes. In 2014, a large randomized controlled trial evaluating the effect of extended lymphadenectomy was presented by a Korean group [18]. Two hundred and forty four patients with resectable pancreatic cancer were enrolled and they were randomly assigned 1:1 to extended resection group or standard resection group. This study also suggested that extended lymphadenectomy with dissection of the nerve plexus did not provide a significant survival benefit compared with standard resection in pancreatic head cancer.

13.3.2 *Laparoscopic Surgery*

Pancreatic cancer surgery has traditionally been carried out as an open procedure, but laparoscopic resections are increasingly being performed. Laparoscopic distal pancreatectomy is increasingly considered a safe and effective option. A systematic review showed superiority of laparoscopic distal pancreatectomy in terms of blood loss, time to first oral intake, and hospital stay [19, 20].

Laparoscopic distal pancreatectomy has, in addition, been performed mainly for benign conditions and there is even scarcer evidence for pancreatic cancer [21]. Especially, little is known about the oncologic outcomes of laparoscopic distal pancreatectomy. A literature suggested that laparoscopic distal pancreatectomy for the patients with pancreatic adenocarcinoma was associated with acceptable long-term oncologic outcomes that median OS was 32 months, and 5-year OS rate was estimated to be 38.2%, respectively [22]. By contrast, laparoscopic pancreatoduodenectomy is a demanding and complex procedure that is not considered standard at present, with increased mortality being a potential issue in low patient volume hospitals [23].

13.3.3 Conversion Surgery/Adjuvant Surgery

A new concept of conversion or adjuvant surgery for initially unresectable pancreatic cancer has recently emerged. Preoperative treatments including chemotherapy and radiotherapy may be proposed to achieve better local tumor control or tumor down-staging with a subsequent potentially resectable tumor. Conversion surgery in this context is defined as surgery after any preoperative therapy aiming to convert unresectable to resectable tumors and to increase microscopic complete tumor resection rates. As today, there is no evidence to perform preoperative treatment for unresectable pancreatic cancer, however, several number of studies were reported for conversion surgery in unresectable pancreatic cancer. Strobel et al. described that gemcitabine-based neoadjuvant therapy for LAPC can achieve high rate of secondary resection (46.7%), and median postoperative survival was greater after resection (12.7 months) than after exploration alone (8.8 months) [24]. Furthermore, Hackert et al. reported that FOLFIRINOX resulted in higher estimated response and resection probabilities (61%) for patients with initially unresectable tumors compared to gemcitabine-based or other regimens [25]. Estimated median survival following resection was 15.3 months for FOLFIRINOX and 8.5 months for exploration alone patients. The period of preoperative treatment can be observation time which allows to find disease progression or poor surgical candidates, and better patient selection. The optimal time for conversion surgery when the tumor should be resected in the process of preoperative therapy is a clinical query. Satoi et al. reported that the appropriate nonsurgical anticancer treatments for better prognosis required over at least 240 days after the initial treatment [26]. To date, data regarding the role of preoperative therapy for unresectable pancreatic cancer from randomized prospective trials are not available. Although a thorough analysis of this group of patients may be hampered by the lack of an accepted patient accommodation for conversion surgery, further careful studies and analyses are critically important to establish the role of conversion surgery.

13.4 Adjuvant Chemotherapy

In 2004, the European Study Group for Pancreatic Cancer 1 (ESPAC-1) trial1 showed that adjuvant chemotherapy (fluorouracil plus folinic acid) had a significant survival benefit in patients with resected pancreatic cancer [27]. In 2005, a large phase III study, CONKO-001 was presented at the American Society of Clinical Oncology (ASCO) Annual Meeting by a German group. CONKO-001 compared a gemcitabine therapy group with a surgery-only group after macroscopically curative resection of pancreatic cancer. CONKO-001 trial showed that adjuvant chemotherapy with gemcitabine not only delayed recurrence, but also improved survival compared with surgery alone. In the study, disease free survival (DFS) was significantly longer in the gemcitabine than in the observation group (median DFS, 13.4 vs. 6.9 months; $P < 0.001$) [28]. Furthermore, OS was also significantly longer in the gemcitabine than in the observation group (median, 22.8 vs. 20.2 months; $P = 0.01$) [29]. In the same way, JSAP-02 study that was the first randomized phase III trial of adjuvant gemcitabine in an Asian population suggested that adjuvant gemcitabine contributed to prolonged DFS in patients undergoing macroscopically curative resection of pancreatic cancer [30]. Recently, several studies showed a survival advantage for patients who received combination systemic chemotherapy in adjuvant setting as compared with patients who received gemcitabine alone. In 2016, JASPAC01 trial showed that superior survival with S-1 compared with gemcitabine [31]. The median OS for patients in the gemcitabine plus S-1 group was 46.5 months (95% CI, 37.8–63.7) compared with 25.5 months (22.5–29.6) in the gemcitabine group (HR = 0.57; 95% CI, 0.44–0.72; $P < 0.001$). Furthermore, ESPAC-4 study also showed that survival with adjuvant chemotherapy with gemcitabine plus capecitabine significantly increased OS compared with gemcitabine alone after resection for pancreatic cancer [32]. The median OS for patients in the gemcitabine plus capecitabine group was 28.0 months (95% CI, 23.5–31.5) compared with 25.5 months (22.7–27.9) in the gemcitabine group (HR = 0.82; 95% CI, 0.68–0.98; $P = 0.032$) (Table 13.2).

Table 13.2 Adjuvant chemotherapy for resected pancreatic cancer

Trial	Year	Regimens	Outcomes
ESPAC-1	2004	FU-RT vs FU vs both vs observation	mOS, 13.9 vs 216 vs 19.9 vs 16.9 mo ($P = 0.05$ for no FU-RT; $P = 0.0009$ for chemo)
JSAP-02	2009	Gem vs observation	mDFS, 11.4 vs 5.0 mo ($P = 0.01$)
CONKO-001	2013	Gem vs observation	mDFS, 13.4 vs 6.7 mo ($P < 0.001$); mOS, 22.8 vs 20.2 mo ($P = 0.01$)
JASPAC01	2016	Gem vs S-1	mOS, 25.5 vs 46.5 mo ($P < 0.0001$)
ESPAC-4	2017	Gem vs gem/cape	mOS, 25.5 vs 28.0 mo ($P = 0.032$)

FU fluorouracil, *RT* radiation, *mOS* median overall survival, *mo* months, *Gem* gemcitabine, *mDFS* median disease free survival, *FOLFIRINOX* 5-fluorouracil, leucovorin, irinotecan, and oxaliplatin, *Cape* capecitabine

The ongoing phase III PRODIGE 24/ACCORD 24 trial comparing adjuvant chemotherapy with modified FOLFIRINOX versus gemcitabine to treat resected pancreatic cancer plans to enroll 490 patients with resected pancreatic cancer and randomize them 1:1 to modified FOLFIRINOX or gemcitabine for 24 weeks; the primary endpoint is progression-free survival. Moreover, other ongoing phase III APACT trial that comparing nab-paclitaxel and gemcitabine vs gemcitabine alone as adjuvant therapy for patients with resected pancreatic cancer aims to demonstrate this benefit in the adjuvant setting, randomly assigning 846 patients with resected pancreatic cancer 1:1 to gemcitabine plus nab-paclitaxel or gemcitabine monotherapy for 24 weeks; the primary endpoint is DFS.

13.5 Neoadjuvant Treatment for Resectable or Borderline Resectable Pancreatic Cancer

The recent improvements of adjuvant therapy were made by the JASPAC 01 and ESPAC4 studies [31, 32]. However, more work is clearly necessary to improve outcomes in the patients with pancreatic cancer after macroscopically curative resection. In order to improve the prognosis, neoadjuvant treatment has drawn attention and several new research are being evaluated. Several trials are ongoing that may clarify whether neoadjuvant chemotherapy or neoadjuvant chemoradiotherapy provides benefits.

13.5.1 Neoadjuvant Chemotherapy

The NEOPAC study is randomized phase II/III trial of neoadjuvant plus adjuvant chemotherapy versus adjuvant alone in resectable pancreatic cancer [33]. The NEOPAC study is randomly assigning patients to neoadjuvant gemcitabine plus oxaliplatin followed by adjuvant gemcitabine, or to adjuvant gemcitabine alone.

The Prep-02/JSAP05 trial is randomized phase II/III trial of neoadjuvant chemotherapy with gemcitabine and S-1 versus upfront surgery for resectable pancreatic cancer. The Prep-02/JSAP05 trial is randomly assigning patients to neoadjuvant gemcitabine plus S-1 followed by adjuvant S-1, or to adjuvant S-1 alone.

The NEONAX trial is randomized Phase II trial of neoadjuvant plus adjuvant or only adjuvant nab-paclitaxel plus gemcitabine for resectable pancreatic cancer. This trial is randomly assigning patients to two cycles of neoadjuvant nab-paclitaxel plus gemcitabine followed by four adjuvant cycles, or to nab-paclitaxel followed by six adjuvant cycles alone.

The SWOG S1505 is randomized phase II/III trial of neoadjuvant chemotherapy with mFOLFIRINOX versus nab-paclitaxel plus gemcitabine for resectable pancreatic cancer. This trial is randomly assigning patients three cycles of neoadjuvant mFOLFIRINOX followed by three cycles of adjuvant mFOLFIRINOX, or to three cycles of neoadjuvant gemcitabine plus nab-paclitaxel followed by three cycles of adjuvant gemcitabine plus nab-paclitaxel.

13.5.2 Neoadjuvant Chemoradiotherapy

The rationale for neoadjuvant chemoradiotherapy in patients with resectable and borderline resectable pancreatic cancer includes several potential benefits [34–37]: down-staging in order to permit resection, improvement in the rate of resection with clear margins, reduction in the incidence of late relapse. Prospective trials of neoadjuvant chemoradiotherapy also are ongoing.

The NEOPA trial is randomized phase III trial of neoadjuvant chemoradiotherapy versus upfront surgery for resectable pancreatic cancer [38]. The NEOPA trial will randomly assign patients to neoadjuvant gemcitabine and concurrent radiation followed by adjuvant gemcitabine, or to adjuvant gemcitabine alone.

The ALLIANCE trial is randomized phase II trial of neoadjuvant chemoradiotherapy versus neoadjuvant chemotherapy for borderline resectable pancreatic cancer [39]. The ALLIANCE trial will randomly assign patients to neoadjuvant modified FOLFIRINOX and subsequent radiation followed by adjuvant FOLFOX, or to neoadjuvant modified FOLFIRINOX followed by adjuvant FOLFOX.

At this moment, there is limited evidence to recommend neoadjuvant treatment for potentially resectable or borderline resectable pancreatic cancer. The above ongoing clinical trials may clarify the significance of neoadjuvant treatment for pancreatic cancer.

13.6 New Treatment

13.6.1 Intraperitoneal Chemotherapy

Positive peritoneal washing cytology (CY) status in patients with resectable pancreatic cancer is defined as M1 disease in the American Joint Committee on Cancer (AJCC) guidelines. Satoi et al. reported that adjuvant chemotherapy did not provide a favorable survival outcome to CY positive patients, and that CY positive patients had poorer prognosis than CY negative patients [40]. To control peritoneal carcinomatosis, new strategy for peritoneal metastasis would be needed. The clinical effects of intraperitoneal paclitaxel in patients with peritoneal metastasis were reported in clinical trials for ovarian cancer [41] and gastric cancer [42]. A phase II study of intravenous and intraperitoneal paclitaxel with S-1 for pancreatic cancer patients with peritoneal metastasis was reported [43]. In the study, 33 patients who were pathologically diagnosed with the presence of peritoneal dissemination or positive peritoneal cytology without other organ metastasis were enrolled. The median OS was 16 months, and the patients who underwent conversion surgery had better prognosis than that of nonsurgical patients.

13.6.2 *Immunotherapy*

Immunotherapy has attracted attention as a novel treatment modality for various carcinoma. Programmed cell death-1 (PD-1) and cytotoxic T-lymphocyte antigen 4 (CTLA-4) are main immune checkpoints activated by tumors to suppress antitumor T-cell responses. Several literatures showed that PD-1–blocking antibodies were used to enhance immunity in solid tumors and obtain clinical responses with safety [44]. Regarding pancreatic cancer, a previous literature suggested that PD-L1 positive patients had a poorer prognosis than the PD-L1 negative patients [45]. Pembrolizumab is one of the immune checkpoint inhibitors that inhibits PD-1 immune checkpoint and has antitumor activity in patients with solid tumors. Pembrolizumab was approved for treatment of patients with non-small-cell lung cancer [46, 47], but was not proven to be safe or helpful in patients with pancreatic cancer. However, recent phase I/II study has reported that gemcitabine, nab-paclitaxel, and pembrolizumab can be safely given to chemotherapy patients with metastatic pancreatic cancer. The prospective randomized phase III trial which proves that pembrolizumab provides better prognosis in pancreatic cancer should be further conducted.

13.7 Conclusion

For the current treatment of metastatic pancreatic cancer, the available chemotherapy regimens including FOLFIRINOX and nab-paclitaxel showed significant improvements in survival, and became considerable options. Although surgery remains the only potentially curative option for resectable disease, newer therapies including gemcitabine/capecitabine and S-1, both of which show superiority to gemcitabine, should be considered new standards of adjuvant treatment after surgery. On the other hand, there are no definitive recommendation and criteria for treatment choice of borderline resectable and locally advanced pancreatic cancer. The role of neoadjuvant therapy remains undetermined. Therefore, there is much room for improvement in all aspects of treatment for pancreatic cancer.

References

1. Kleeff J, Korc MAM. Pancreatic cancer. Nat Rev Dis Primers. 2016;2:16022.
2. Rahib L, Smith BD, Aizenberg R, et al. Projecting cancer incidence and deaths to 2030: the unexpected burden of thyroid, liver, and pancreas cancers in the United States. Cancer Res. 2014;74:2913–21.
3. Bockhorn M, Uzunoglu FG, Adham M, et al. Borderline resectable pancreatic cancer: a consensus statement by the International Study Group of Pancreatic Surgery (ISGPS). Surgery. 2014;155:977–88.

4. Tempero MA, Malafa MP, Behrman SW, et al. Pancreatic adenocarcinoma, version 2.2014 featured updates to the NCCN guidelines. J Natl Compr Cancer Netw. 2014;12:1671–80.
5. Tempero MA, Malafa MP, Al-Hawary M, et al. Pancreatic adenocarcinoma, version 2.2017, NCCN clinical practice guidelines in oncology. J Natl Compr Cancer Netw. 2017;15:1028–61.
6. Burris HA III, Moore MJ, Andersen J, et al. Improvements in survival and clinical benefit with gemcitabine as first-line therapy for patients with advanced pancreas cancer: a randomized trial. J Clin Oncol. 1997;15:2403–13.
7. Moore MJ, Goldstein D, Hamm J, et al. Erlotinib plus gemcitabine compared with gemcitabine alone in patients with advanced pancreatic cancer: a phase III trial of the National Cancer Institute of Canada Clinical Trials Group. J Clin Oncol. 2007;25:1960–6.
8. Conroy T, Desseigne F, Ychou M, et al. FOLFIRINOX versus gemcitabine for metastatic pancreatic cancer. N Engl J Med. 2011;364:1817–25.
9. Ueno H, Ioka T, Ikeda M, et al. Randomized phase III study of gemcitabine plus S-1, S-1 alone, or gemcitabine alone in patients with locally advanced and metastatic pancreatic cancer in Japan and Taiwan: GEST study. J Clin Oncol. 2013;31:1640–8.
10. Von Hoff DD, Ervin T, Arena FP, et al. Increased survival in pancreatic cancer with nab-paclitaxel plus gemcitabine. N Engl J Med. 2013;369:1691–703.
11. Chandrasegaram MD, Goldstein D, Simes J, et al. Meta-analysis of radical resection rates and margin assessment in pancreatic cancer. Br J Surg. 2015;102:1459–72.
12. Bilimoria KY, Bentrem DJ, Ko CY, et al. National failure to operate on early stage pancreatic cancer. Ann Surg. 2007;246:173–80.
13. Nimura Y, Nagino M, Takao S, et al. Standard versus extended lymphadenectomy in radical pancreatoduodenectomy for ductal adenocarcinoma of the head of the pancreas. J Hepatobiliary Pancreat Sci. 2012;19:230–41.
14. Pedrazzoli S, DiCarlo V, Dionigi R, et al. Standard versus extended lymphadenectomy associated with pancreatoduodenectomy in the surgical treatment of adenocarcinoma of the head of the pancreas: a multicenter, prospective, randomized study. Lymphadenectomy Study Group. Ann Surg. 1998;228:508–17.
15. Yeo CJ, Cameron JL, Sohn T, et al. Pancreaticoduodenectomy with or without extended retroperitoneal lymphadenectomy for periampullary adenocarcinoma: comparison of morbidity and mortality and short-term outcome. Ann Surg. 1999;229:613–24.
16. Riall TS, Cameron JL, Lillemoe KD, et al. Pancreaticoduodenectomy with or without distal gastrectomy and extended retroperitoneal lymphadenectomy for periampullary adenocarcinoma - part 3: update on 5-year survival. J Gastrointest Surg. 2005;9:1191–206.
17. Farnell MB, Pearson RK, Sarr MG, et al. A prospective randomized trial comparing standard pancreatoduodenectomy with pancreatoduodenectomy with extended lymphadenectomy in resectable pancreatic head adenocarcinoma. Surgery. 2005;138:618–30.
18. Jang J-Y, Kang MJ, Heo JS, et al. A prospective randomized controlled study comparing outcomes of standard resection and extended resection, including dissection of the nerve plexus and various lymph nodes, in patients with pancreatic head cancer. Ann Surg. 2014;259:656–64.
19. Venkat R, Edil BH, Schulick RD, et al. Laparoscopic distal pancreatectomy is associated with significantly less overall morbidity compared to the open technique: a systematic review and meta-analysis. Ann Surg. 2012;255:1048–59.
20. Mehrabi A, Hafezi M, Arvin J, et al. A systematic review and meta-analysis of laparoscopic versus open distal pancreatectomy for benign and malignant lesions of the pancreas: it's time to randomize. Surgery. 2015;157:45–55.
21. Sulpice L, Farges O, Goutte N, et al. Laparoscopic distal pancreatectomy for pancreatic ductal adenocarcinoma. Ann Surg. 2015;262:868–74.
22. Sahakyan MA, Kim SC, Kleive D, et al. Laparoscopic distal pancreatectomy for pancreatic ductal adenocarcinoma: long-term oncologic outcomes after standard resection. Surgery. 2017;162:802–11.
23. De Rooij T, Lu MZ, Steen MW, et al. Minimally invasive versus open pancreatoduodenectomy: systematic review and meta-analysis of comparative cohort and registry studies. Ann Surg. 2016;264:257–67.

24. Strobel O, Berens V, Hinz U, et al. Resection after neoadjuvant therapy for locally advanced, "unresectable" pancreatic cancer. Surgery. 2012;152:S33–42.
25. Hackert T, Sachsenmaier M, Hinz U, et al. Locally advanced pancreatic cancer. Ann Surg. 2016;264:457–63.
26. Satoi S, Yamaue H, Kato K, et al. Role of adjuvant surgery for patients with initially unresectable pancreatic cancer with a long-term favorable response to non-surgical anti-cancer treatments: results of a project study for pancreatic surgery by the Japanese Society of Hepato-Biliary-Pan. J Hepatobiliary Pancreat Sci. 2013;20:590–600.
27. Neoptolemos JP, Stocken DD, Friess H, et al. A randomized trial of chemoradiotherapy and chemotherapy after resection of pancreatic cancer. N Engl J Med. 2004;350:1200–10.
28. Oettle H, Post S, Neuhaus P, et al. Adjuvant chemotherapy with gemcitabine vs observation in patients undergoing curative-intent resection of pancreatic cancer. JAMA. 2007;297:267–77.
29. Oettle H, Neuhaus P, Hochhaus A, et al. Adjuvant chemotherapy with gemcitabine and long-term outcomes among patients with resected pancreatic cancer. JAMA. 2013;310:1473.
30. Ueno H, Kosuge T, Matsuyama Y, et al. A randomised phase III trial comparing gemcitabine with surgery-only in patients with resected pancreatic cancer: Japanese Study Group of Adjuvant Therapy for Pancreatic Cancer. Br J Cancer. 2009;101:908–15.
31. Uesaka K, Boku N, Fukutomi A, et al. Adjuvant chemotherapy of S-1 versus gemcitabine for resected pancreatic cancer: a phase 3, open-label, randomised, non-inferiority trial (JASPAC 01). Lancet. 2016;388:248–57.
32. Neoptolemos JP, Palmer DH, Ghaneh P, et al. Comparison of adjuvant gemcitabine and capecitabine with gemcitabine monotherapy in patients with resected pancreatic cancer (ESPAC-4): a multicentre, open-label, randomised, phase 3 trial. Lancet. 2017;6736:1–14.
33. Heinrich S, Pestalozzi B, Lesurtel M, et al. Adjuvant gemcitabine versus NEOadjuvant gemcitabine/oxaliplatin plus adjuvant gemcitabine in resectable pancreatic cancer: a randomized multicenter phase III study (NEOPAC study). BMC Cancer. 2011;11:346.
34. Sho M, Akahori T, Tanaka T, et al. Pathological and clinical impact of neoadjuvant chemoradiotherapy using full-dose gemcitabine and concurrent radiation for resectable pancreatic cancer. J Hepatobiliary Pancreat Sci. 2013;20:197–205.
35. Sho M, Akahori T, Tanaka T, et al. Optimal indication of neoadjuvant chemoradiotherapy for pancreatic cancer. Langenbecks Arch Surg. 2015;400:477–85.
36. Takahashi H, Ohigashi H, Gotoh K, et al. Preoperative gemcitabine-based chemoradiation therapy for resectable and borderline resectable pancreatic cancer. Ann Surg. 2013;258:1040–50.
37. Takahashi H, Ohigashi H, Gotoh K, et al. Preoperative gemcitabine-based chemoradiation therapy for resectable and borderline resectable pancreatic cancer. Ann Surg. 2016;262:e103.
38. Tachezy M, Gebauer F, Petersen C, et al. Sequential neoadjuvant chemoradiotherapy (CRT) followed by curative surgery vs. primary surgery alone for resectable, non-metastasized pancreatic adenocarcinoma: NEOPA- a randomized multicenter phase III study (NCT01900327, DRKS00003893, ISRCTN82191749). BMC Cancer. 2014;14:411.
39. Katz MHG, Ou F-S, Herman JM, et al. Alliance for clinical trials in oncology (ALLIANCE) trial A021501: preoperative extended chemotherapy vs. chemotherapy plus hypofractionated radiation therapy for borderline resectable adenocarcinoma of the head of the pancreas. BMC Cancer. 2017;17:505.
40. Satoi S, Murakami Y, Motoi F, et al. Reappraisal of peritoneal washing cytology in 984 patients with pancreatic ductal adenocarcinoma who underwent margin-negative resection. J Gastrointest Surg. 2014;19:6–14.
41. Armstrong DK, Bundy B, Wenzel L, et al. GOG 172 Intraperitoneal cisplatin and paclitaxel in ovarian cancer. N Engl J Med. 2006;354:34–43.
42. Ishigami H, Kitayama J, Kaisaki S, et al. Phase II study of weekly intravenous and intraperitoneal paclitaxel combined with S-1 for advanced gastric cancer with peritoneal metastasis. Ann Oncol. 2009;21:67–70.

43. Satoi S, Fujii T, Yanagimoto H, et al. Multicenter phase II study of intravenous and intraperitoneal paclitaxel with S-1 for pancreatic ductal adenocarcinoma patients with peritoneal metastasis. Ann Surg. 2017;265:397–401.
44. Brahmer JR, Tykodi SS, Chow LQ, et al. Safety and activity of anti-PD-L1 antibody in patients with advanced cancer. N Engl J Med. 2012;366:2455–65.
45. Nomi T, Sho M, Akahori T, et al. Clinical significance and therapeutic potential of the programmed death-1 ligand/programmed death-1 pathway in human pancreatic cancer. Clin Cancer Res. 2007;13:2151–7.
46. Garon EB, Rizvi NA, Hui R, et al. Pembrolizumab for the treatment of non–small-cell lung cancer. N Engl J Med. 2015;372:2018–28.
47. Reck M, Rodríguez-Abreu D, Robinson AG, et al. Pembrolizumab versus chemotherapy for PD-L1–positive non–small-cell lung cancer. N Engl J Med. 2016;375:1823–33.

Index

H. Yoshiji, K. Kaji (eds.), *Alcoholic/Non-Alcoholic Digestive Diseases*,
https://doi.org/10.1007/978-981-13-1465-0

MIX
Papier aus verantwortungsvollen Quellen
Paper from responsible sources
FSC® C105338

FSC
www.fsc.org

If you have any concerns about our products,
you can contact us on
ProductSafety@springernature.com

In case Publisher is established outside the EU,
the EU authorized representative is:
Springer Nature Customer Service Center GmbH
Europaplatz 3, 69115 Heidelberg, Germany

Printed by Libri Plureos GmbH
in Hamburg, Germany